Case Studies in Biomedical Rese

Basic Bioethics
Glenn McGee and Arthur Caplan, editors

Case Studies in Biomedical Research Ethics

Timothy F. Murphy

The MIT Press
Cambridge, Massachusetts
London, England

This book was set in Sabon by Achorn Graphic Services, Inc.
Printed and bound in the United States of America.

Library of Congress Cataloging-in-Publication Data

Murphy, Timothy F., 1955–
  Case studies in biomedical research ethics / Timothy F. Murphy.
    p. cm. — (Basic bioethics)
  Includes bibliographical references and index.
  ISBN 0-262-13437-3 (hc : alk. paper) — ISBN 0-262-63286-1 (pbk. : alk. paper)
  1. Medical ethics—Case studies. 2. Bioethics—Case studies. 3. Medical ethics—Research—Case studies. 4. Bioethics—Research—Case studies. I. Title. II. Series.

R724.M876 2003
174.2—dc22
                                                          2003060799

Printed on recycled paper.

10 9 8 7 6 5 4 3 2 1

Contents

Series Foreword

We are pleased to present the ninth volume in the series Basic Bioethics. The series presents innovative book-length manuscripts in bioethics to a broad audience and introduces seminal scholarly manuscripts, state-of-the-art reference works, and textbooks. Such broad areas as the philosophy of medicine, advancing genetics and biotechnology, end of life care, health and social policy, and the empirical study of biomedical life will be engaged.

Glenn McGee
Arthur Caplan

Acknowledgments

Ethical questions about research are embedded not only in the pages of history but also in the most important research initiatives of the day. Despite the richness of sources, this casebook took time to take form. Some of these cases had their first hearing during a 1999–2001 research ethics seminar for scholars in the Chicago area. I led this group as the principal investigator of a National Institutes of Health (NIH) grant. These scholars gathered monthly to identify key issues in research ethics and to develop projects appropriate to their own institutions. In the 1990s the Clinton administration and Congress set aside funds to advance instruction in research ethics, and the NIH initiative that followed was more than necessary to the development of this book. Without that grant, I would only have dabbled with these cases as class handouts; I certainly would not have gathered them together in this form. Courses must have useful materials, and it is my hope that this casebook will be useful to existing courses and spur the development of new ones.

For either writing cases or providing materials that served as the basis for cases, I thank Robert Binstock of Case Western Reserve University; Robert Folberg of the University of Illinois at Chicago; Mark Waymack of Loyola University of Chicago; and Kenneth Pimple, Vicki Field, and Peggy Sundemeyer of Indiana University. B. Taylor Bennett at the University of Illinois at Chicago took the time to discuss research uses of animals. I also very much want to thank Gregory E. Pence of the University of Alabama at Birmingham for his help in identifying cases that deserved inclusion. During his very busy first year in medical school, Jonah Murdock sought me out for conversations, and these led to his role as an assistant to the project; for identifying some cases to be included I thank him. I am also grateful to Alfred Pach III for a memorable conversation that led to one hypothetical case. Several University of Illinois at Chicago physicians who participated in an ethics seminar offered counsel about the Introduction: John Davis, Arnold M. Eiser, Asra Khan, and Mary Lou Schmidt. As I brought the manuscript to completion, the Institute for Ethics at the American Medical Association offered me its resources when I served there as visiting scholar. I appreciate the resources and conversations generously given during that time. Anonymous reviewers for The MIT Press also offered challenging comments on the early draft, and I appreciate their assiduous advice. I thank Carrie Golus for editorial assistance over and above the call of duty. She rescued the manuscript after an office-temp from hell left it in an electronically despoiled state.

Many thanks also go to John F. Harris for tolerating stretches of self-absorption, patches of ill temper, monologues posing as conversation, and disruptions of vacations as this manuscript lurched ahead. I wish I could promise that they won't happen again.

Despite the assistance I have had with this book, I offer a sincere demurral of responsibility for any errors. I acknowledge any problems in the representation of these cases as my own responsibility.

I gratefully acknowledge permissions given to use materials taken from the following publications:

Lawrence K. Altman, *Who Goes First? The Story of Self-Experimentation in Medicine* (Berkeley: University of California Press, 1998).

Edward J. Huth, "Irresponsible Authorship and Wasteful Publication," *Annals of Internal Medicine* 1986 (104): 257–259.

Steve Jones, "Genetics in Medicine: Real Promises. Unreal Expectations: One Scientist's Advice to Policy Makers in the United Kingdom and the United Sates," Milbank Memorial Fund, 2000, p. 17.

Nancy M. P. King, Gail E. Henderson, Jane Stein, eds., *Beyond Regulations: Ethics in Human Subject Research* (Chapel Hill, NC: University of North Carolina Press, 1999).

Dorothy Nelkin, "The High Cost of Hype," in Ruth Ellen Bulger, Elizabeth Heitman, Stanley Joel Reiser, eds., *The Ethical Dimensions of the Biological Sciences* (Cambridge: Cambridge University Press, 1993), pp. 270–277.

Mary Briody Mahowald, *Genes, Women, Equality* (New York: Oxford University Press, 2000).

Jonathan D. Moreno, *Undue Risk: Secret State Experiments on Humans* (New York: W. H. Freeman, 1999).

F. Barbara Orlans, Tom L. Beauchamp, Rebecca Dresser, David B. Morton, John Gluck, *The Human Use of Animals: Case Studies in Ethical Choice* (New York: Oxford University Press, 1998).

Christobel Saunders, Michael Baum, Joan Houghton, "Consent, Research, and the Doctor-Patient Relationship," in Raanan Gillon, ed., *Principles of Healthcare Ethics* (Chichester: John Wiley & Sons, 1994), pp. 457–469.

Robert M. Veatch, Amy Haddad, *Case Studies in Pharmacy Ethics* (New York: Oxford University Press, 1999).

Preface

The book is intended as a text for instruction in biomedical research ethics. Cases are its heart and can be used as resource in a variety of settings. Taken as a collection, the cases introduce some key episodes and debates in biomedical research ethics. They are as short as they can reasonably be to convey their core elements. Some cases simplify events and debates, but in each I have tried to convey an accurate sense of historical events, even if they offer only a window on the past rather than a complete vista. Each case has a brief introduction that offers context for the case and the issues it raises. For the most part, the cases are drawn from historical records and from articles in the scientific and bioethics literature. A note identifies source materials for cases quoted or adapted from published works. Identified sources can be used for further research in the area. Other cases are purely hypothetical, drawn up to illustrate particular kinds of problems; they are always identified as fictional.

Most cases are drawn from the biomedical sciences, although I could not help including a few salient ones from the social sciences. By the overwhelming focus on biomedical research, I do not mean to slight the social sciences that make essential contributions to knowledge. It strikes me, however, that full consideration of cases from the social sciences probably requires a book in its own right, and I have not attempted to fold two projects into one.

As an instructor with many years in front of a classroom, I have rarely found questions from teacher's manuals very useful. They can be stilted and limiting, the pedagogical equivalent of a lesson plan left for use by a substitute teacher hastily called in at the last minute. I have found that armed with sufficient information and left to their own devices, discussants are quick to raise many questions that open a topic for meaningful analysis. I have supplied study questions at the end of each case but hope that these are used as triggers for discussion, not as ends in themselves. At the end of the Introduction I have identified some core questions that may be profitably applied to research in general.

This book will not be all things to all people, but it can educate and spur discussion about key events and debates in research ethics, a history with its own full share of dubious and ill-conceived ventures. It is not enough to look at this history as a voyeur; it is important to engage this history with an eye to identifying principles and practices that can help guide biomedical research toward respectful and humane treatment of subjects and toward consistency in matters of social justice.

As an editorial note, let me say that in presenting the case materials in this format, some minor changes have been made while adapting original materials. For example, when quoting materials directly, I have broken some long paragraphs into smaller ones. Other editorial modifications are similarly minor.

Cases by Chapter

Case Studies in Biomedical Research Ethics

Introduction

A prominent anthology of bioethics devotes one-third of its considerable length to ethical theory before going on to analyze issues of abortion, gene therapy, death and dying, and so on.[1] This is not terribly surprising. Many such anthologies offer a substantial tour of ethics theory before turning to specific topics. A great deal of analysis in ethics is given to self-examination, to consideration of whether its methods and procedures are sound. Ethics sometimes goes a long theoretical way before coming to judgment on a given topic.

That said, at the present time there are many accepted concepts and practices in research ethics. They involve codes of ethics, core principles, formal regulations, and oversight mechanisms used to evaluate the morality of research in life sciences. This is not to say that all matters are fully settled as a matter of social or political consensus: many ethical issues are still under live debate. But it is to say that identifiable starting points are available from which to begin an ethical analysis of biomedical research.

Oversight of Research

Some ethical issues in medicine, such as abortion and euthanasia, have lineages that reach back to the earliest organized efforts at healing. By comparison, research ethics—in the sense of a sustained analysis of motives for, process of, and social effects of biomedical research—is of comparatively recent vintage. For the vast majority of human history, very few efforts were made to articulate and implement standards for research involving people and animals. Formal protections for human research subjects did not move forward in an unbroken and linear way.[2] On the contrary, that process progressed in fits and starts. Sometimes unwritten professional standards worked to protect subjects from undue risk and to secure their voluntary participation. Sometimes researchers saw the need for more formal standards. In 1932, for example, the United States Navy initiated some requirements for informed consent in its research projects. These early developments were the exception rather than the rule, and in some instances there were jaw-dropping lapses in professional conduct. Researchers around the globe sometimes used humans without their knowledge or consent: death, disease, and profound insults to dignity were the result. Ultimately, these scandals contributed to the development of formal codes that had no precedent in medicine.

In many ways, contemporary research ethics begins with the scandals of experimentation conducted in the World War II era. During the Nazi regime, researchers exposed subjects to extreme cold, pressure, diseases, and unproved therapies. They also killed humans to obtain biological specimens.[3] People used in these experiments were chosen from the imprisoned, the weak, and the reviled. In preparation for the 1947 trials against the responsible parties, United States physicians Andrew Ivy and Leo Alexander drew up for the court (and this was the first time it had been done) formal statements they said defined ethical standards observed in research with human beings.[4] In its judgments, the court used the principles to identify what it called permissible medical experiments. This text has become known as the Nuremberg Code. (See appendix A.)

During the trials, the accused doctors argued that their experiments were no different from those being conducted by other German physicians or by United States physicians for that matter. They also maintained that they were not violating specific professional standards. They said that for the period in which they stood accused no international standards specified the difference between licit and illicit experiments with human beings. In fact, this argument had some validity. It was only in late 1946, as the trials were being planned, that the American Medical Association followed Dr. Ivy's lead and adopted formal ethical advisories with regard to the conduct of research with human beings. During the trial, Dr. Ivy stated that whereas formal guidelines for research were not written down anywhere, "They were understood only as a matter of common practice."[5] Most accused Nazis were found guilty over their protests.

The misuse of humans in research occurred not only under the Nazis, who were committed to the genocide of Jews, homosexuals, Gypsies, and others they found objectionable. The military government of imperial Japan also sponsored far-ranging and lethal experiments that involved vivisection, battlefield injuries, hypothermia, and exposure to lethal infectious diseases. The subjects were citizens—men, women, and children—in occupied China who were more or less chosen at random for their horrendous fates.[6]

Despite Dr. Ivy's view that widespread consensus existed in the medical community about how researchers should treat human subjects, the reality was that even in the United States abuses were begging for correction, for example, the infamous Tuskegee syphilis study that began in 1932 (see chapter 1).

Despite the war crimes trials, the Nuremberg Code had an uneventful reception in the United States. It was not immediately disseminated and incorporated into United States standards and law. In a telling incident, in 1953 the Secretary of Defense did promulgate the Nuremberg Code as a guide to research dealing with atomic, biological, and chemical warfare.[7] This decision was treated, however, *as a state secret,* and it was kept classified and released only to key parties. Military decisions are frequently treated as secrets, and in this case the secrecy may have been a matter of habit. It might also have been influenced by a wish to hide biological and chemical warfare programs. As might be expected, because the directive was kept secret, the principles of the Nuremberg Code were not widely disseminated and fully incorporated in military research. In fact, it was not until 1975 that the decision to use the code as a guide to research was declassified and made general knowledge.

By 1975, the World Medical Association had already adopted its ethical advisory with regard to biomedical research. The association is a group whose members are from medical associations around the world. It adopted its World Declaration of Helsinki in 1964. (Several modifications have been made since that time. See appendix B for the entire text.) This document has become a major focal point when evaluating the ethics of particular studies.

The United States began to define and implement a system of systematic regulations from the 1950s and 1960s on. It started in major federal departments, sometimes with parallel developments in the military.[8] The process was, again, sporadic. Some physicians resisted adopting formal codes because they felt that codes would interfere excessively with the patient-physician relationship. Ultimately, research scandals provided the political impetus to institute formal protections for research subjects, to complete the work begun with the Nuremberg Code. In 1966, Henry K. Beecher published a widely discussed article in the *New England Journal of Medicine,* identifying twenty-two examples of objectionable research taken from medical journals of the day.[9] In one instance, researchers exposed twenty-six newborns to multiple X-rays to learn whether they had reflux of urine from the urethra to the bladder. These babies experienced no such problem, and Beecher worried that the extensive radiation exposure might cause problems later in their lives. In another example, researchers conducting bronchoscopies—an examination of the air passageways through a tube—added another component to that process: they inserted a special needle through the windpipe into the left atrium of the heart in patients who did and those who did not have cardiac disease. Beecher thought it was clearly wrong to expose patients with no heart problems to this new technique that had unknown hazards. He did not identify individuals involved in these studies, as his goal was not to accuse or to sanction, but to increase awareness of the need for greater protection of research subjects. Although his report did not lead to immediate change, it did sensitize the medical community to the protection of subjects.

One long-running U.S. research study is worth mentioning in detail. In 1932 the government initiated an observational study of syphilis in African-American men that did not end until a journalist brought it to national attention in 1972.[10] The point was to learn whether syphilis had a different pathological course in black men than in white men. Approximately 623 African-American subjects with and without the disease were recruited from the poor, rural county of Macon, Georgia. They would be followed throughout their lives and autopsied at death to determine how the disease had progressed. During the decades, infected subjects were not treated, even though an effective therapy had become widely available. In addition, no member of the original control group who contracted syphilis during the course of the study was treated. The researchers, in fact, actively conspired with physicians in the area to prevent these subjects from obtaining treatment. Moreover, they actively lied to the men about their condition. In 1972, embarrassed officials brought the study to an end, but its repercussions remain to this day. The specter of the Tuskegee study is never far from analysis of African-American health care in this country.[11]

Coupled with other scandals, such as intentional exposure of institutionalized children to hepatitis at Willowbrook,[12] the Tuskegee study helped build the political will to move the United States toward a systematic and formal regulation of research standards. In 1974, Congress approved the National Research Act and established an important advisory body: the National Commission for the Protection of Human Subjects of Biomedical and Behavioral Research. It also required that all research funded by the Department of Health, Education, and Welfare receive prior review and approval from local review committees. The National Research Act did not extend to all federal research. Military research was not covered, and privately funded research was exempt as well. Nevertheless, the Act did establish the system of Institutional Review Boards (IRBs) now in place, and that is no small accomplishment. These IRBs are local committees that determine whether certain standards of subject protection are met before research may commence.

The work of the National Commission also led to the extremely influential 1978 *Belmont Report,* which identified three main concepts by which to evaluate the ethics of research.[13] These guiding concepts have been the subject of much analysis and criticism. They do not exhaust the entirety of ethical analysis, but they do offer an excellent starting point from which to evaluate the motives for, the process of, and the social impact of research. The *Belmont Report* identified three key concepts as guides for research: respect for persons, beneficence, and justice. Respect for persons asserts the importance of recognizing persons as their own decision makers and protecting those who are unable to make decisions for themselves. Researchers must offer potential subjects adequate information about the project, ensure that subjects comprehend the information, and ensure the voluntary nature of participation. The concept of beneficence asserts the importance of protecting the welfare of subjects. It requires researchers to offer a meaningful balance of risks and benefits. Justice refers to an equitable distribution of risks and benefits across groups. Researchers must ensure that no particular group is favored in access to and distribution of research benefits. They must also ensure that no group is exposed excessively to risks of research or denied its benefits. It falls to IRBs to implement these concepts as they are embodied in federal regulations. The core functions of an IRB are described briefly in chapter 1. The *Code of Federal Regulations* may be consulted for a more complete description of the nature and scope of IRB responsibilities.[14]

It is unlikely that current standards for the oversight of research will remain static. They will continue to respond to social pressures, including scandals that might come to light. To improve the system now in place, a number of advisory bodies have proposed many changes to mechanisms of oversight. In 2001, the National Bioethics Advisory Commission recommended that Congress put in place a system that required *all* research in the United States to be reviewed under the authority of a single agency.[15] The commission also made a variety of recommendations about the responsibilities of IRBs. Many other bodies and independent academic commentators have also suggested ways in which to improve the oversight of research in the United States.[16] Whether these recommendations will be acted on remains to be seen. In the meantime, the nature and scope of oversight will remain a matter of continuing debate. This debate will not only look at individual research projects themselves but will continue to assess the tools by which ethical analysis does its work.

It should be mentioned that ethical analysis of research with animals has followed a historical trajectory of its own. Some of the issues at stake in animal research are discussed in the introduction to chapter 8.

Looking at the Past through the Lens of Today

It should be understood that some of the cases in this book took place at a time when there were no formal requirements that projects must undergo review and receive approval from an independent body. While sensitivity to research ethics was evident in some quarters, a robust sense of subject protection had not fully filtered through the scientific community.

One point to keep in mind while looking at the past is the distinction between *wrong-doing* and *blameworthiness*. It can be tempting to condemn all researchers in the past as blameworthy because their work failed in some way to meet standards now in place. While many studies failed ethical tests we would apply today and are therefore examples of wrongdoing, not all the researchers are blameworthy in the way researchers today might be. Some of them may be judged less harshly because of mitigating factors, such as factual ignorance, cultural ignorance, evolution in moral understanding, and organizational indeterminacy.[17] Factual ignorance refers to information researchers at that time could not have had and on which they could not be expected to act. Cultural ignorance refers to moral sensitivities that a culture as a whole might not have. For example, it is difficult to see individual researchers as blameworthy for a particular problem, for example, using prisoners for experimentation, when their practice was very much of a piece with the views of their time. The evolution of moral understanding refers to changes in the way we interpret morality. It can be inappropriate to hold researchers to standards that are only fully developed much later. Finally, organizational indeterminacy refers to unclear responsibility within an organization or group. It can sometimes be inappropriate to blame particular individuals for moral failures that are more properly speaking failures of their organizations as a whole. It is often more useful to study the past in order to guide the present than to try and affix degrees of blameworthiness to people long since dead.

Case Study in Ethics

It is not enough these days simply to publish case studies without some explanation. Some critics contend that the study of cases seriously short-changes ethical theory. Tod Chambers has argued that ethicists should stop writing cases because the format does not permit the kind of critical depth that ethics requires and ought to pursue.[18] According to this viewpoint, cases cover up more than they reveal. For example, they can wrongly emphasize the priorities at stake (there might be another perspective from which to view the problem), skew relevant details (the author may have a vested interest in representing the issue in a particular way), and establish hierarchies of authority about who is entitled to what (the case may reflect a decision-making process that should itself be called into question). If all these things were true, morality would certainly evolve as critics maintain: as unconnected and random epiphanies. The danger looms that case analysis would be essentially anecdotal. Despite this criticism, I believe many things justify the use of cases.[19] Case analysis is at heart *casuistry,* an evaluation of particular situations in light of generally held principles or beliefs. This method has nothing inherently quibbling or evasive about it, despite disparaging use of the term casuistry. The work of case analysis is not the only work to be done in ethics, but it does a great deal of the heavy lifting.

In the main, case analysis moves from details to consideration of more general ethical precepts and principles. The depth of the analysis resides in locating a particular case along a spectrum of paradigmatic ones whose resolution is clear in one way or another. John Arras rightly pointed out that to "know" bioethics is to know these key cases and to appreciate how to situate new ones beside them. I do not find that criticisms of casuistry and case study cut against them in any mortal way. Cases are instruments of exploration. One does not need an alternative text to ask whether something about the presentation of issues—about the implicit urgency, detail, or authority structure—should be called into question. The conceptual force that one brings to the case, rather than the form itself, is the measure of its success. Neither does one require a novel-like depiction of a problem in order to ask whether there is something self-serving about its details and the mechanisms available for resolution. I suppose that one could say that poems would be more successful if they were more like novels and offered more description and context. But a poem's form has a value of its own and it does not necessarily short-change larger questions of meaning.

Case analysis can acutely capture the way in which moral dilemmas *are dilemmas,* circumstances in which values are set against one another. A case, especially one that offers discussants a narrative guide in the form of a protagonist, antagonist, supporting cast, and the need for resolution, can do this very well. For example, it can raise problems that occur when researchers are torn between competing designs for a study: one design might offer faster answers while another might protect its subjects from certain risks. Which way to go? A single case can be a good starting point for a discussion of competing models—and values—in the design of clinical trials.

Case analysis can also provide historical education of a kind. Cases that draw on historical examples can serve as summaries of key events and landmark decisions that shape the practice of research ethics today. I do not mean that they can take the place of searching historical analysis that examines issues fully in their times and contexts, but they can stimulate historical awareness in circumstances in which one is expecting "only" ethics. In other words, cases can be a spur to historical analysis as discussants ask how present-day practices and policies have come to be the way they are.

That the threshold for entry into cases is low does raise concerns that case analysis may lend itself to easy pontifications, hasty treatment, and overdrawn conclusions. The excesses of easily formed opinions are not, of course, the problem of case analysis alone. More expansive texts and theoretical backgrounds cannot protect against lazy assumptions or hasty conclusions. Ultimately, it is not the case itself, and especially not its length, but the quality of analysis that will matter most in casuistry.

Nothing about case analysis excludes systematic ambition in ethical analysis. It can be tempting to solve an immediate ethical problem, such as sexual harassment in the research environment, without raising larger concerns about professional conduct more generally. One does not have to invoke an overarching theory of workplace standards to stop one lecherous scientist from putting graduate students in compromising situations. Needless to say, it would certainly be preferable to ensure that educational settings as a whole are free from sexual misconduct, but nothing in the case approach prevents anyone from raising exactly that broader question. In that sense, it is the imagination and initiative of those doing the study that set limits to the reach of the analysis.

John Arras has said that casuistry "always risks a facile accommodation to the prejudices of the day" because it relies on settled convictions and common responses to cases.[20] For example, if ten misogynistic commentators examine a case involving exclusion of women from research trials, it is likely that they will carry their antipathy toward women into that analysis. But it is unclear that this worry cuts against the method of casuistry in a significant way since the prejudices of the day will be in place no matter what kind of moral reasoning discussants invoke. People who invoke an elaborate theoretical structure for ethical analysis can be just as misogynistic as anyone else. Ethical analysis is only as good as its tools, and that remains true whether its text is a short, telegraphed communication or a leisurely stroll though textual hill and contextual dale.

Rather than assuming that ethical analysis is meaningful only it if relies on the machinery of a complete and overarching theory, the question of the depth of analysis should itself be a matter for discussion. Case analysis can be useful in achieving low-level resolutions precisely because fundamental agreement at all levels is not necessary for each and every ethical difficulty. For example, people who disagree about the value of some research can reach consensus about its funding, not because they agree about its value but because they respect *the process* that leads to decisions about funding. It can be respect for others' views that brings about a morally defensible conclusion to a problem rather than agreement at a deeper philosophical level. One should not expect from a subject—and that includes ethical analysis—any more degree of precision than it can sustain.

A final concern is that case analysis does not worry enough about the status of its outcomes. Do its resolutions impose obligations on others? For example, suppose that four discussants are examining a case of plagiarism by a senior scientist. They may poke, prod, and probe the case for all its details and come to a conclusion about the charges and evidence. What standing does their analysis have? Does their conclusion represent anything more than their own opinions writ large? Is there any way in which their conclusion should be binding on others? Does their conclusion represent a moral perspective that could be generalized? To come to a conclusion, case analysis does not seem to require that a proposed resolution is binding on others. But neither does it stand in the way of asking whether this resolution does, in fact, have force outside their agreement. It may well be that no universally binding precept is necessary to resolve a single episode of plagiarism. By the same token, people doing case analysis can also bring into question the moral standing of their methods and conclusions.

To ensure that some aspect of the case does not take analysis in a wrong direction, certain cautionary questions should be asked: (1) Is the problem one that requires ad hoc resolution or something more ambitious? (2) Does the case reveal problems with accepted ethical norms, laws, or policies? (3) Are ethical precepts or principles at conflict with one another in formulating a response to this case, and if so, how should that conflict be sorted out? Which precepts or principles ought to take priority and why? (4) Does any aspect in the representation wrongly influence the way in which the case might be discussed or resolved? For example, are key facts left undisclosed, or is the authority of the participants used to the disadvantage of anyone else? In the end, the conceptual force brought to bear can overcome inherent weaknesses of the form.

Ethical Analysis in Research—Guiding Questions

Several points of analysis should be addressed in evaluating the ethics of research, no matter what specific moral theory is invoked or what kind of research involved. These are the motives for, the process of, and the social impact of research. The relative value of these points will vary depending on the circumstances of the issue under consideration. Some relevant questions are as follows.

Motives for Research

1. What values are represented by the research?
2. What is the justification for this area of research compared with other possible areas?

3. Does anything about the proposed research misapprehend problems and their potential solutions?

4. What priority and funding should be given to the research given competing lines of research?

5. Does sponsorship, through funding or personalities involved, influence the nature and significance of the research? If so, how might undue influences be eliminated or controlled?

Process of Research

1. Does the process of research bring important values or principles into conflict?

2. Is the process somehow in conflict with stated goals?

3. Is the research sufficiently justified in terms of conducting it with animals? adults? children? people in compromised or vulnerable states?

4. Does a justifiable rationale exist for including and excluding various subjects?

5. Does the research have equity of access?

6. Are risks fairly distributed across human subjects?

7. Are benefits fairly distributed across human subjects?

8. Does the research comply with accepted standards of conduct?

9. What degree of oversight, if any, is required during the research or the period of its influence?

Social Impact of Research

1. Do effects of this research establish or reinforce some kind of inequity, for example, prejudicial treatment or discrimination?

2. Do the effects alter existing social compacts about privacy, social institutions, social opportunities, or democratic process in fundamental ways?

3. Are possible findings so potentially divisive that the research should not be conducted?

4. How should the results be integrated into society?

5. What challenges to the legal system might follow?

6. What standard ought to apply to the social distribution of benefits that come out of research?

Many questions in research ethics do not have the sort of flashy allure found in life-and-death medicine. Nonetheless, the issues are among the most important in biomedicine today. They are important because they affect tens of thousands of people a year who participate in clinical trials, not to mention the many millions of animals used around the world. At stake are the health, well-being, and dignity of these participants. At stake are outcomes that determine medical treatment, health policies, food supplies, and economic gain. Also at stake are values and goals of society, as commitments are made to the study of a particular area and forgoing other areas of study. Biomedical science is not the only domain that poses questions of this kind for humanity, but it is perhaps the domain over which we have the greatest opportunity for reflection and choice. We are obliged, then, to raise and resolve many ethical questions about motives for, process of, and social effects of research. Beyond analysis of these particular focal points, it is also important to reflect on the meaning of research projects, what they signify for political compacts, for the meaning of communal social life, and even for human nature itself. It is to be kept in mind, of course, that human nature may not refer to a fixed, static reality but to what can be summoned from human beings. And that is perhaps the key starting point for ethical analysis in research: what are we asking from ourselves in the name of science?

References

1. Helga Kuhse, Peter Singer, eds., *A Companion to Bioethics* (Oxford: Blackwell, 1998).

2. A presidential advisory committee described the early emergence of research ethics standards in the United States, and should be consulted for a detailed examination of the period between 1940 and 1974: Advisory Committee on Human Radiation Experiments, *Final Report of the Advisory Committee on Human Radiation Experiments* (New York: Oxford University Press, 1996).

3. Andrew C. Ivy, "Nazi War Crimes of a Medical Nature," *Federation Bulletin* 1947 (33): 133–146. George J. Annas, Michael A. Grodin, eds., *The Nazi Doctors and the Nuremberg Code: Human Rights in Human Experimentation* (New York: Oxford University Press, 1992).

4. Advisory Committee on Human Radiation Experiments, *Final Report of the Advisory Commission on Human Radiation Experiments* (New York: Oxford University Press, 1996), pp. 75–78.

5. *Final Report of the Advisory Committee*, p. 78.

6. Sheldon H. Harris, *Factories of Death: Japanese Biological Warfare, 1932–1945, and the American Cover-up* (New York: Routledge, 1994).

7. *Final Report of the Advisory Committee*, pp. 56–61.

8. *Final Report of the Advisory Committee*, pp. 45–73.

9. Henry K. Beecher, "Ethics and Clinical Research," *New England Journal of Medicine* 1966 (274): 1354–1360.

10. James H. Jones, *Bad Blood: The Tuskegee Syphilis Experiment*, rev. ed. (New York: Free Press, 1993).

11. See Susan M. Reverby, ed., *Tuskegee's Truth: Rethinking the Tuskegee Syphilis Study* (Chapel Hill: University of North Carolina Press, 2000).

12. David J. Rothman, Sheila M. Rothman, *The Willowbrook Wars* (New York: Harper & Row, 1984).

13. National Commission for the Protection of Human Subjects of Biomedical and Behavioral Research, *The Belmont Report: Ethical Principles and Guidelines for the Protection of Human Subjects of Research.* Washington, DC: Department of Health, Education, and Welfare, 1978.

14. The Code of Federal Regulations is the compilation of federal law. The section dealing with IRBs can be found at 45 C.F.R. 46.

15. National Bioethics Advisory Commission, *Ethical and Policy Issues in Research involving Human Participants* (Washington, DC: National Bioethics Advisory Commission, 2001).

16. Office of the Inspector General, *Institutional Review Boards: A Time for Reform* (Washington, DC: Dept. of Health and Human Services, 1998).

17. I borrow these factors from the Advisory Committee on Human Radiation Experiments, *Final Report of the Advisory Committee on Human Radiation Experiments* (New York: Oxford University Press, 1996), pp. 121–123.

18. Tod Chambers, "Why Ethicists Should Stop Writing Cases," *Journal of Clinical Ethics* 2000 (11): 206–211. See also Tod Chambers, *The Fiction of Bioethics: Cases as Literary Texts* (New York: Routledge, 1999).

19. I owe much of this discussion to my reading of John D. Arras, "A Case Approach," in Helga Kuhse, Peter Singer, eds., *A Companion to Bioethics* (Oxford: Blackwell, 1998), pp. 106–114.

20. Arras, p. 113.

1

Oversight and Study Design

Introduction

In the United States and elsewhere, an independent ethics committee must review and approve many research projects that involve human beings. For example, the National Institutes of Health may offer grant support for research on diabetes prevention in adolescents, but the study would have to be reviewed in advance by a committee because of its use of federal money. The use of radioactive substances in research with humans, although not necessarily sponsored by the federal government, would also require review because it involves regulated substances. Local committees doing this work have different names around the world, and in the United States, Institutional Review Boards (IRBs) evaluate whether a research project is designed in a way that protects the rights and welfare of its subjects. Beyond the review required by government regulations, a good deal of research with human beings is overseen by IRBs because universities and other institutions sometimes extend federal policy to all research regardless of the funding source. In other words, they apply one set of rules to all research.

Not all research that involves human beings requires review and approval of IRBs. For example, teachers may wish to evaluate the benefits of textbooks, curricula, and teaching strategies in primary school. This does not require review and approval. The same is true of privately funded research that is not intended to bring a product to market; for example, studies of weight-loss products.

Responsibilities of IRBs offer a useful starting point for the ethical evaluation of research. This is not to say that these responsibilities are the only areas to analyze. It is to say that they capture some of the most important features of the analysis. In reviewing the responsibilities of an IRB, it is well worth wondering whether their structure and functions are equal to their task. In other words, it should not be assumed that the existing mechanism of oversight is completely adequate. Knowing the responsibilities of an IRB will help provide key concepts necessary to discuss the cases in this chapter.

One word of caution is in order: some of the cases in this chapter took place before it was formally required that researchers receive approval for their projects. Some hospitals and other institutions did, early on, set up ad hoc ethics committees to address particular concerns.[1] Most of the time, however, no review and approval by an independent committee were required before starting research with humans.

Responsibilities of IRBs

Federal regulations require that IRBs be composed in a certain way and carry out certain functions as they review research protocols. Primary areas of concern for the boards are membership diversity and expertise, informed consent of subjects, subject selection with special attention to vulnerable populations, monitoring safety, and confidentiality.[2]

Membership Diversity and Expertise   The issue of membership is tied to the board's core functions. Federal regulations specify a minimal number of members (five), in addition to requirements with regard to community representation, diversity, and nonscientific practitioners, among others.[3] At least one member of the IRB should not be affiliated with the sponsoring institution. Membership should be diverse with regard to race, gender, and cultural backgrounds. It should also be attuned to the community in which the research is being done. The board must meet other membership requirements when certain populations are involved; prisoners, for example. Furthermore, no IRB may consist of members of a single profession. One member should represent a nonscientist point of view, and there must also be at least one scientist. All members should have enough expertise to be able to understand whether the institution has the capacity to undertake the research. Some member must be conversant with relevant professional and legal standards. If the IRB lacks expertise to pass judgment on a particular research protocol, it may invite others to offer their counsel, though these outside experts may not vote on the protocol. The regulations also work to control conflict of interest. Members who have research pending before the IRB may not participate in the review of this research, except to offer information.

Informed Consent   IRBs are charged to ensure that research participants know that they are involved in research and that they have the right to participate or not. Specifically, the board has the duty to ensure that subjects know what kind of research they are involved in and how long it will last, what risks and discomforts it might involve, and what benefits are involved, if any.[4] This informed consent process should occur in language that is comprehensible to the subjects.

For medical interventions, the IRB must see to it that researchers disclose to subjects alternatives to participating in the research. If there is compensation for participation, the board must make sure that this is disclosed. Furthermore, it should ensure that the informed consent process discloses whether compensation is available if the study injures them, and where they might turn for treatment. The IRB must also ensure that informed consent makes it clear that subjects have the right to withdraw from the study at any time without penalty or loss of benefits they would otherwise have. The board must require researchers to tell subjects that they have rights as participants and where to look for further information. It must also ensure adequate documentation of subjects' consent to participate.

Subject Selection   IRBs must see that principles of fairness govern selection of research subjects.[5] They must ensure that no prejudicial reason exists for including or excluding people from a study. For instance, physicians might draw subjects from their patients, but there should be no reason apart from scientific needs as to why some are included and others are excluded. The IRBs must assess whether and to what extent a project is relying on subjects simply because of their availability, compromised positions, or ease of management. For example, researchers might wish to study prostate cancer in a Veterans Affairs hospital simply because such a hospital would have a good number of men being treated for this condition. However, to rely on veterans' hospitals exclusively as a source of subjects is to skew the distribution of risks and benefits to a single group, rather than to distribute them more widely across all men with prostate cancer. By attending to such matters, the IRB can rule out exploitation of an easily available population as well as systematic exclusion from potential medical benefits.

Vulnerable Populations   As an additional requirement when considering the selection of subjects, federal regulations spell out duties for research involving certain vulnerable populations: pregnant women, children, and prisoners.[6] Limitations are in place with regard to the kind of research that may be conducted with these populations and the way in which studies may be approved. For example, researchers who intend to study prisoners are ordinarily limited to projects that are of interest to prison populations themselves, as opposed to using prisoners for random purposes. Research is regulated to protect children from risks unless those risks are offset by some potential benefit to the children, although there can be some exceptions (45 CFR 46, Sec. 407). Research with pregnant women is similarly restricted. Review boards that routinely deal with research with vulnerable populations are required to have representation in their membership of people familiar with these groups. Thus they can make an informed evaluation of the nature, risks, and benefits of a particular study.

Monitoring   The IRB is responsible for evaluating risks and benefits of a study and ensuring that researchers have appropriate mechanisms in place to identify and treat risks that emerge.[7] For example, if subjects receiving a drug that places them at risk of vasculitis (a potentially serious inflammation of blood vessels) it is appropriate for the IRB to insist on a reasonable schedule of clinic visits to identify and treat this condition should it develop. Over and above ensuring that researchers conduct adequate monitoring during a study, IRBs must review each study at least once a year and more often if significant risks are involved.

Confidentiality   Research participation can jeopardize participants in a variety of ways. For example, if a young man does not want it known in his community that he has AIDS, he will not want to participate in a study that would make this common knowledge. Protecting confidentiality will protect this man's status in the community. Once in the study, confidentiality becomes important for other reasons. People may not be inclined to offer their actual views or behave in the way they would normally if they believe that the research could expose them in some way. It is the IRB's job to ensure that researchers do what they can to protect participants from risks related to disclosure of their involvement in a study.[8] In practical terms, boards must ensure that researchers take from subjects only information that is important to the study. They must also oversee the way in which data are recorded, analyzed, and stored. If an IRB believes that some aspect of data management puts subjects in jeopardy, it may refuse to approve the study.

Study Design

The most important scientific goal of a study is to contribute to knowledge. Failure to meet this goal has led to many regrettable occurrences. In the worst of these, people were subjected to harmful interventions that did not make significant contributions to science, such as studies carried out by Nazi and Imperial Japanese researchers, which also involved subjects against their will. The ability of a study to make a contribution to science is one of the first conditions of ethical research. If research cannot offer meaningful results it is hardly ethical to ask people to waste time participating, let alone exposing themselves to risks.

At the very least, therefore, researchers should have sufficient knowledge of their field to ensure that their work will make a new contribution and not duplicate existing knowledge. Research is not based on a single model. As a matter of protecting subject rights and welfare, ethical analysis has to take into account the variety of study designs and how different ones might carry different risks and benefits.

Kinds of Studies   Some studies are *observational*: a researcher observes the course of events in an area. A sociologist may want to describe rituals involved in providing medical care in emergency departments. The researcher therefore describes health care workers as they go about their work. A pathologist may wish to describe the way in which a viral infection progresses to symptoms and disease, again, without altering phenomena under study. Other studies involve the study of *an intervention* on those phenomena. A pediatrician may wish to study the effects of counseling in reducing childhood aggression in the classroom, a psychiatrist may wish to study the effects of a new antipsychotic drug. In these instances, the goal is to identify how things unfold or move forward as a result of the intervention. Their goal is to isolate the effects of the intervention from other factors that might influence outcomes.[9]

Some studies are carried out for *nontherapeutic* reasons. Here, the intervention is not intended to have a particular benefit to the subject. For example, a researcher may wish to study whether a new skin ointment causes allergic reactions in humans. In applying the ointment, the researcher has no intention of helping the subject. In *therapeutic research*, it is hoped that the intervention will benefit the subject. The same researcher might wish to know whether that ointment helps treat insect bites. Obviously, the degree of risk in studies can vary from virtually nonexistent to life-threatening, depending on what the study involves and how it is designed.

Inclusion and Exclusion Criteria   Researchers use *inclusion* and *exclusion criteria* to identify people they believe will be the best subjects. In the study of a drug treatment for kidney disease, inclusion criteria might stipulate symptoms required for someone to be eligible to participate. If, for some reason, this drug could not be studied safely in children, exclusion criteria would rule out their involvement. Other exclusion criteria might point to ways in which a subject should be excluded once it is under way. For example, a subject who became too ill to continue might be withdrawn from the experimental drug. Inclusion and exclusion criteria are often excellent points for analyzing access and equity in subject selection.

Placebos   Many people respond to an encounter with a physician or other health professional as if they have received a beneficial therapy, even if they have not. In these instances, *expectation of benefit* produces improvement through psychological means and not through actual treatment.[10] This response pattern is known as the *placebo effect*. When studying one or more medical interventions, researchers must take some measures to rule out the placebo effect so that the actual merit of the intervention can be identified clearly. When the placebo effect is known to be present, researchers will design the study to have two arms: the active arm and the placebo arm. Subjects in the active arm receive the intervention and those in the placebo arm receive an inert intervention. When the study is done, researchers can compare the effect of the intervention against that of the placebo. The use of placebos is not deceptive if subjects agree to enter the study knowing they may not receive the active treatment.

Not all trials require a placebo, and in some instances placebos should not be used for moral reasons. For example, if a pharmaceutical company wants to introduce a new drug to treat severe high blood pressure, that drug could be tested against a placebo. But it is morally problematic to ask people who are already taking a drug that controls high blood pressure to stop taking *that drug* and enter into a trial in which they will receive either *a drug of unknown risk and benefit* or *no drug at all*. For this reason, it is a generally accepted moral requirement that experimental agents and devices are tested against existing, accepted treatments. Some researchers argue, however, that certain studies should be entitled to use placebos if there is a pressing reason to do so.

Randomization and Blinding   For a variety of reasons, some studies are *randomized* and *blinded*. Randomization refers to enrollment by chance into various arms of the study. A researcher may wish to evaluate the merits of a new drug to treat kidney disease against an existing one. To protect against the placebo effect, and to ensure that nothing about subject selection will influence the outcome, the researcher will assign subjects by chance to receive either the new agent or existing treatment. This can be done by various means, such as computer-generated assignments.

Blinding refers to keeping the assignments—whether receiving the new drug or the existing one—from the participants. In a *single-blind study,* subjects do not know what treatment they are receiving; researchers do know. In a *double-blind study* neither subjects nor researchers know who is receiving the drug and who is receiving the alternative intervention or placebo. In double-blind, placebo-controlled studies, the sponsor supplies researchers with drugs and placebos in coded batches. The placebo will ordinarily appear identical to the drug formulation. In case of medical emergency, provisions allow for *unblinding* a study so that a physician can know how to treat a subject who becomes ill.

Equipoise   When is it justified to use human beings for experimental research? Part of the answer is to be found in *equipoise,* which refers to a collective state of uncertainty about the best way to treat a particular condition.[11] This uncertainty is due to competing beliefs and absence of definitive information on the topic. To justify exposing humans to risks, it should be expected that the study will help undercut this uncertainty. If physicians have reason to think that an available treatment is highly effective in treating a particular condition, they have little justification to ask their patients to enroll in a study of an untested drug. However, for some conditions no such existing treatment may be available or researchers may think that a new drug is far superior to existing ones. For example, data from animal studies may hint that a new agent could be far more effective than current ones. Or the new drug might only have to be taken once a day rather than four times. In any case, at the point of equipoise, uncertainty clouds which course of treatment might be better. It would undermine a physician's fiduciary responsibility to ask patients to enroll in a study that is conducted without strong reasons for thinking that the new agent is at least as good as an existing one. It is a kind of informed uncertainty that justifies asking subjects to enroll in research studies.

Clinical Care and Research Requirements

In one sense some biomedical interventions carried out by physicians are experimental but do not require review and approval. A degree of flexibility is necessary in clinical practice to accommodate the specific needs of patients, and for this reason it is not desirable to require that physicians seek review and approval for *all* departures from accepted professional standards. For example, physicians may judge that it is important to vary recommended dosages of a particular drug. Or surgeons may decide to manage a particular intestinal repair in a way not well studied or well established. In 1978, the *Belmont Report* tried to protect a domain of clinical innovation while at the same time suggesting that, at an early point, innovations should be subjected to formal study. It concluded, "When a clinician departs in a significant way from standard or accepted practice, the innovation does not, in and of itself, constitute research. The fact that a procedure is 'experimental' in the sense of new, untested or different, does not automatically place it in the category of research. Radically new procedures of this description should, however, be made the object of formal research at an early stage, in order to determine whether they are safe and effective. Thus, it is the responsibility of medical practice committees, for example, to insist that a major innovation be incorporated into a formal research project."[12] Obviously, introduction of clinical innovations can raise important questions about the nature and scope of risks patients are asked to accept.

References

1. Advisory Committee on Human Radiation Experiments, *Final Report of the Advisory Committee on Human Radiation Experiments* (New York: Oxford University Press, 1996).

2. Robert J. Levine, *Ethics and Regulation of Clinical Research*, 2nd ed. (New Haven, CT: Yale University Press, 1988).

3. 45 CFR 46 Sec. 407.

4. 45 CFR 46 Sec. 416.

5. 45 CFR 46 Sec. 111.

6. 45 CFR 46 Subparts B, C, D.

7. 45 CFR 46 Sec. 111.

8. 45 CFR 46 Sec. 111.

9. For further information about study design, see Sana Loue, *Textbook of Research Ethics: Theory and Practice* (Dordrecht: Kluwer Academic / Plenum Publishers, 1999), pp. 217–239.

10. Howard Brody, *Placebos and the Philosophy of Medicine: Clinical, Conceptual, and Ethical Issues* (Chicago, IL: University of Chicago Press, 1980).

11. Benjamin Freedman, "Equipoise and the Ethics of Clinical Research," *New England Journal of Medicine* 1987 (317) 3: 141–145.

12. National Commission for the Protection of Human Subjects of Biomedical and Behavioral Research, *The Belmont Report: Ethical Principles and Guidelines for the Protection of Human Subjects of Research* (Washington, DC: Department of Health, Education, and Welfare, 1978).

1.1

The Tuskegee Syphilis Studies

It is important for medicine to know the way in which a disease progresses in order to identify symptoms and develop effective treatments. It is also important to know whether disease manifests differently according to age, gender, and race. At the start of the project discussed below, the specific effects of syphilis in "Negro males" were not well studied. Research that began as an attempt to answer questions about the course of the disease has become one of the enduring hallmarks of unethical research in the United States.

In 1932, the US Public Health Service enrolled African-American men from Macon County, Alabama, home of the Tuskegee Institute, in a study of the natural history of syphilis. The site was chosen because Macon County had one of the highest rates of syphilis in the nation. Approximately 623 men were recruited by offers of free medical examinations and blood tests. Approximately half of them had syphilis at the beginning of the study, although none of them was told that fact. Because of poverty in the county and limited health services, it is unlikely that these men would have had access to treatment in any case. During the course of the study, some of the men in the control group would contract syphilis as well.

At that time there was medical uncertainty about the effects of syphilis in African-Americans. Other groups had been studied, but concern arose that the disease progressed differently depending on race. It was believed that in African-Americans syphilis had more effect on the cardiovascular system than on the central nervous system. Questions also concerned the value of available treatments, including suspicion that some were worse than the disease itself. The researchers wanted to study the men to the time of death and conduct autopsies to provide definitive data. During the decades that followed, the men were studied at various points. They underwent medical examinations, blood tests, and lumbar punctures to evaluate neurological aspects of the disease. They received these interventions without cost, were given free rides to the examinations, and were treated for minor ailments, and their families received a small burial stipend. From time to time, the researchers published various findings. During the late 1940s and early 1950s, effective treatments for syphilis became widely available; however, none was offered to the men in the study. In fact the names of these men were circulated among physicians in the region to ensure that they would not receive treatment.

In 1969, criticism began to surface, and a Public Health Service committee met to determine whether or not to continue the study. This committee recommended that the study go forward, although it did indicate that some subjects might be treated medically on a case-by-case basis. In 1972, a critic who was not satisfied with this outcome brought the study to the attention of Associated Press journalist Jean Heller. Her newspaper reports provoked another review, and the study was formally brought to an end in November 1972.

Study Questions

1. How important are the research questions underlying this study? Could this information have been obtained in another way? How many subjects were put at risk by this study?

2. To what extent do you think that this study went on for as long as it did because of the subjects who were involved? What factors made them vulnerable?

3. In 1997, President Clinton formally apologized to seven subjects who were still living. What elements do you think should be in a formal apology to such survivors?

Adapted from James H. Jones, *Bad Blood: The Tuskegee Syphilis Experiment*, rev. ed. (New York: Free Press, 1993). See also Susan Reverby, ed., *Tuskegee's Truths: Rethinking the Tuskegee Syphilis Study* (Chapel Hill: University of North Carolina, 2000) and Fred D. Gray, *The Tuskegee Syphilis Study: The Real Story and Beyond* (Montgomery, AL: New South, 1998).

1.2

Desperate Measures

Patients with life-threatening and debilitating illnesses are often desperate to find treatments. In the 1980s, this was especially true when AIDS was not well studied with regard to causes and treatments. The case below describes the actions of one twenty-six-year-old man in a trial of azidothymidine (AZT). To his mind, desperation justified not only cheating to be accepted into the clinical trial but also swapping experimental pills with another subject. The case raises interesting questions about the ethics of enrolling dying or very ill subjects in clinical trials.

Paul Sergios, age 23 years, began to experience symptoms of AIDS in 1983, well before there were treatments. Almost immediately, he began to pursue remedies, only to come up empty-handed. He turned to underground pharmacies operated by people with AIDS and their advocates. These pharmacies would often make compounds they thought were promising, even if these drugs were not proved to be useful.

In 1986, Sergios located a phase II trial of AZT being conducted through the AIDS Clinical Trial Group. It was a double-blind, placebo-controlled trial in which half the subjects would receive the drug, and the rest would receive an inert sugar pill. Phase II trials are designed to learn whether a drug has an effect on a disease; a phase III trial would be required to learn whether that effect, if any, offers benefit to the patient in terms of controlling symptoms.

Criteria for entry into the trial were that subjects have a certain level of CD4 cells; thrush (an infection of mucosal tissues), weight loss, or swollen lymph nodes; and nonresponsiveness to certain immune-response skin tests. Sergios met the first two criteria. The third was in doubt. At the clinic, a nurse administered four needle-sticks into Sergios's *left* forearm and wrote a number on each puncture site that corresponded to the antigen injected there. If inflammation appeared at the sites, it meant that the immune system was still functioning and Sergios would be excluded from the study. In fact, he showed some immune response. Sergios was despondent: he was basically too healthy to get in, but he was certain that the drug could buy him time. To be accepted into the study, a friend wrote four numbers on Sergios's *right* forearm, and he presented this arm to the clinic nurse, who saw no immune response and declared him eligible.

Once in the study, Sergios knew that he might receive active drug or placebo. He took his pills to a friend, a "midnight chemist" (i.e., a self-trained chemist working outside the law), in hopes of finding out which pills he had received. The friend was unable to tell him, but he suggested that Sergios and another subject in the study swap half their pills. That way, they each increased their chances of getting at least some of the active drug. Sergios was reluctant, thinking that swap would be immoral. The chemist saw things another way: "Immoral?" he asked, "What about their twisted morality in giving half of us a sugar pill for a year or two in order to see how fast we go to our deaths while others get a drug that could potentially save their lives? Not only that—this study prohibits us from taking certain drugs to prevent opportunistic infections. The odds are stacked against us." Sergios and his friend swapped half their pills during the course of the trial.

Study Questions

1. What is the reason for having exclusion criteria in a research trial, and do you think this study was justified in using them?

2. Why is it ethical (or unethical) to ask people to enter a placebo-controlled study like the one described?

3. Do you think that the deceptions carried out by the subjects were justified? Could researchers have worked with the subjects to avoid the deceptions?

Adapted from Paul A. Sergios, *One Boy at War: My Life in the AIDS Underground* (New York: Knopf, 1993), pp. 81–85.

1.3

Surgical Innovation and Research

The boundary between innovation and research in surgery is often blurry. Even for the same procedure, what a surgeon will do varies with different patients. Moreover, surgeons often look to their own clinical judgment rather than to clinical trials to gauge what is in a patient's best interest. In fact, some surgeons resist randomized clinical trials, even though these trials are considered the gold standard of medical evidence elsewhere. Some of the reasons for this resistance are described below.

Surgeons sometimes maintain that their work does not lend itself to randomized clinical trials. They contend, for example, that a good series of cases can be more useful in determining the value of a particular technique or strategy. Indeed, surgical techniques may be diffused throughout the medical community before they have been fully evaluated in formal research trials. If trials are under way, techniques may be adopted before the results are fully compiled and evaluated.

Some commentators hold that clinical trials almost always create nonrepresentative samples of patient populations and that results are of limited value. Others point out that clinical trials are expensive, cumbersome, and difficult to complete. They believe that trials take too long, that various options can become available to surgeons during that time that make studies obsolete. Some surgeons do not like being locked into particular techniques or management strategies. In fact, the main complaint about randomized surgical trials is that they undercut the ability of surgeons to make recommendations based on their knowledge and experience. This is all the more true, some surgeons believe, for patients who have life-endangering or profoundly disabling conditions.

Study Questions

1. Federal regulations allow physicians to use an innovation that has not been studied in formal research as long as it is intended to benefit an individual patient. Why are regulations designed this way?

2. How convincing is the allegation that the value of surgical interventions can be ascertained in ways that do not rely on randomized clinical trials?

3. The *Belmont Report* recommends that clinical innovations be studied in a formal way as soon as practical. At times, however, a surgical approach to disease becomes quickly established as the standard of care without such study. When this happens, it becomes difficult to conduct studies because researchers do not want to deprive patients of the benefit of the new approach. Do you think a series of case studies reporting success with a technique is sufficient to meet the expectations of the *Belmont Report* for formal study?

Adapted from Joel E. Frader, Donna A. Caniano, "Research and Innovation in Surgery," in Laurence B. McCullough, James W. Jones, Baruch A. Brody, eds., *Surgical Ethics* (New York: Oxford University Press, 1988), pp. 216–241.

Artificial Hearts: The Need for Review

Federal regulations draw a distinction between therapeutic innovations and formal research. Therapeutic innovations are those steps physicians take to manage the diseases of individual patients, whereas research is intended to clarify matters of fact in a general way. Since the 1960s and 1970s, considerable interest has been expressed in designing an artificial heart. The case below raises important questions about early interventions with an artificial heart.

In April 1969, Dr. Denton Cooley of the Texas Heart Institute implanted an artificial heart of his design into Haskell Karp, who was in terminal heart failure. A potential donor of a human heart had arrived at the Heart Institute but not in time to allow its use. Karp's condition had deteriorated too quickly to pursue that option.

Because the chair of the relevant committee was not available at the time, Cooley went ahead with the artificial heart transplantation without review by the U.S. Public Health Service, whose review and approval at that time was required for all new medical devices. In any case, Cooley claimed that he did not need permission, because the intervention was intended as therapy and not an experiment.

Michael DeBakey, another physician who had been working on an artificial heart, was furious that Cooley had gone ahead with this transplant. He had not known that Cooley had obtained access to his own research and had hired some of DeBakey's former staff to help develop a competing artificial heart.

Karp survived for only three days after the operation. After his death, his wife filed suit, alleging malpractice. She said she and her husband had not understood that he had so little hope of returning to a normal life, even though he had signed consent forms describing considerable risks of the intervention. She claimed they were not sufficiently advised about the likelihood of her husband being in so much pain, having so much nausea, and being comatose for a great deal of the time. In addition, neither she nor her husband had understood that the main intent of the intervention was to test the feasibility of the device in human beings.

The court dismissed this lawsuit, perhaps in part because DeBakey did not testify. In 1971, Cooley implanted another artificial heart, again without asking a relevant body for review or permission. Once again, he said that he did so because of the emergency faced by the patient. This patient died two days after the operation.

Study Questions

1. It is one thing to read a list of possible complications of surgery, and it is another thing to understand what they would mean if they actually occur. What means might be used to help patients and research subjects to a better understanding of the risks that might occur during the course of treatment?

2. Is it convincing to maintain that no review or approval of a mechanical heart is necessary because without it a patient is in immediate danger of death?

3. Is it fair to ask patients at imminent or serious risk of death if they are willing to accept the risks of an unproved device? Are patients in such a condition ever in a position to refuse?

Adapted from Gregory E. Pence, *Classical Cases in Medical Ethics* (New York: McGraw-Hill, 1990), pp. 299–301.

Access to Nonapproved Drugs

Since 1962 the United States has required that researchers receive approval from the Food and Drug Administration (FDA) to test drugs for safety and effectiveness in humans. To receive this approval, researchers must complete an investigational new drug application. They must describe the composition of the drug, preclinical testing of its safety (including animal studies), the protocol of planned testing, qualifications of the investigators, and provisions for obtaining informed consent of research subjects. Once approved, researchers may conduct phase I trials to identify safe dosage ranges, toxicity, and various pharmacological data in a small number of subjects; phase II trials to study the effect of the drug in small numbers of subjects; and phase III trials to study the safety and clinical value of the drug in larger numbers of subjects. As these trials proceed, the FDA reviews the data to determine whether to approve commercial use of the drug. As can be imagined, this process can be long and laborious. People often want access to drugs before they have undergone this process. The FDA has tried to strike a balance between scientific rigor and compassion toward people with life-threatening illnesses. There are, however, critics on both sides of this policy: that it undermines science or that it is unsympathetic to people who are at risk of death.

Azidothymidine (AZT), was developed in 1964 and was intended as a cancer treatment, but proved not to be beneficial. In 1984 and 1985, the drug showed some effectiveness against the human immunodeficiency virus (HIV) in laboratory experiments. In 1985 its manufacturer, Burroughs-Wellcome, filed an investigational new drug (IND) application with the FDA, and a randomized, placebo-controlled trial in 282 people with AIDS began in February 1986. After six months, nineteen subjects in the placebo arm had died, compared with only one in the drug arm. Faced with these results, researchers concluded that it would be unethical to continue the study. At the same time, they acknowledged that they had no way of knowing whether the drug would have any beneficial long-term effects or risks. At that point, they were merely trying to determine whether it had a measurable effect. Despite the fact that the death rate in the placebo arm was higher than that in the active arm, it might be that AZT delayed death only for a short period of time or might show dangerous side effects later on.

This study had a significant impact on opinion about research trials, especially for people with life-endangering diseases. To respond to such emergencies, the FDA now makes provision for a treatment IND that allows distribution of a drug during final phases of testing and review, before all the data are in. No people receiving the drug under this circumstance are studied in research trials.

Advocates maintain that people with such serious diseases should be allowed to accept greater risks when their lives are at stake. Critics worry that administering experimental drugs under treatment INDs may broaden their use and undermine the scientific gold standard of testing that is necessary to determine actual clinical benefits and risks over the short and long term.

Study Questions

1. What ethical concerns are associated with releasing a drug before formal evaluation shows that it is both safe and efficacious?

2. In what way does nearness to death or having a severe disorder justify access to an experimental drug?

3. Would it be fair to require that anyone receiving an experimental drug under a treatment IND also participate in a formal evaluation of its effect? In other words, people would have access to the drug only if they agreed to serve as research subjects. Would this imply a measure of forced participation?

Adapted from Baruch Brody, *Ethical Issues in Drug Testing, Approval, and Pricing: The Clot-Dissolving Drugs* (New York: Oxford University Press, 1995), pp. 163–172.

Off-Label Use of Drugs

Physicians commonly prescribe drugs for purposes other than those approved by the FDA. This is called off-label use. Although the drug is approved for a specific use, physicians may rely on their clinical judgment to use it for other purposes. Malpractice standards are the check-and-balance system on this use rather than formal oversight by a government agency. Widespread off-label prescribing of a drug may lead to a call for formal studies of its risks and benefits. In these cases, the lines between clinical use and research sometimes become blurry.

Dr. Valerian, a urologist, had been involved in the research on Viagra that led to FDA approval as a treatment for male impotence. During this time he became convinced that Viagra could also benefit women suffering from decreased tumescence during sexual stimulation.

In fact, Dr. Valerian began to prescribe Viagra for women soon after the FDA approved it for men. These women reported benefits analogous to those reported for men. In time, Dr. Valerian routinely prescribed Viagra for women who had difficulties with vaginal stimulation. Over two years his patient records seemed to indicate clearly that the drug helped women in approximately the same proportion as it helped men. It also had similar limitations. For example, diabetic women were infrequently helped by it, as is the case with men. After three years, Dr. Valerian believed he might be able to publish the results of his treatment.

Study Questions

1. In what sense, if any, was Dr. Valerian conducting research when he first began prescribing Viagra to women?

2. In what way would it be appropriate—if at all—for Dr. Valerian to use data from his medical records in a research report? Do you believe he should ask his patients' permission to use their records in this way?

1.7

When Does Research Begin?

It is sometimes unclear when research begins, namely, when a researcher progresses from having an idea to planning a formal study. For example, researchers may simply begin investigating a particular topic before realizing that they want to conduct a complete study of it. In the case below, a university initiated a misconduct inquiry when it believed a researcher had not received the appropriate approval to go forward with his investigation.

In 1995, John Wilmoth met Christian Mortensen at a retirement home. Wilmoth, who was a demographer at the University of California at Berkeley, had heard Mortensen was 112 years old. Wilmoth believed that it would be interesting to confirm this man's age, because he would be among the world's oldest men. He thought he might conduct interviews to add a human-interest angle to articles he would write on human longevity.

Wilmoth consulted Mortensen's legal guardian and his doctor, who agreed that such contact would be good for the older man's social stimulation. At the first meeting, Wilmoth asked Mortensen questions such as, "Gee, how old are you? When were you born? What are your happinesses in life?" The two continued to chat frequently over a few months. Then Wilmoth contacted his university's IRB because he wanted to give Mortensen some mental agility tests. On learning of the meetings with Mortensen, the IRB accused Wilmoth of failing to report contact with a vulnerable human subject, and in 1996 the university began a misconduct investigation. Wilmoth saw himself as a victim of "regulatory mania." In 1998, Mr. Mortensen died at 115 years of age.

Study Questions

1. In what way, if any, did Professor Wilmoth's conversations put Mr. Mortensen at risk? Was there any benefit from the conversations?

2. Do you think Wilmoth should have sought review and approval for his initial conversations with Mortensen?

3. After six months of investigation, a committee of three Berkeley professors cleared Wilmoth. One committee member expressed surprise that the investigation could have been raised on such grounds. How might a university avoid unprofitable investigations such as this in the future?

Adapted from Christopher Shea, "Don't Talk to the Humans," *Lingua Franca*, Sept. 2000, pp. 27–34.

Surrogate End Points in Research

When testing drugs, it is important to know whether they slow morbidity and mortality. However, it is not desirable to let studies go on so long that subjects become sick and die. For this reason, researchers may try to identify subclinical markers to track the emergence of disease. For example, changes in immunological responses or various cell counts can show whether a drug is having an effect, even before people have symptoms or face the risk of death. These markers are known as surrogate end points, and they stand in for actual disorders and death in the hope that researchers can measure result of a drug's benefit more quickly. It is important that surrogate end points be strongly correlated with actual clinical conditions so that they can be used as indicators of the intervention's effect.

One study took as its focus the effect of AZT when administered either immediately after HIV infection is diagnosed or later when symptoms of AIDS began to appear. In particular, researchers were interested in the effects of this drug when these people had very low counts of CD4 cells. Subjects who received the drug usually showed an immediate increase in CD4 cell counts. After participating in the trial for one year, however, subjects were significantly different in the way they were progressing toward disease, with those receiving the drug being less likely to have major symptoms than subjects receiving placebo. After three years, no significant difference was evident between the groups with regard to either symptoms or survival rates. Critics were quick to point out that measurement of CD4 cells did not correlate with improved protection from illness or survival in the long run.

Study Questions

1. What are surrogate end points, and why are they desirable? Did this study use a meaningful surrogate end point?

2. What benefits to subjects were identified after one year of the study? Did they remain after three years? Were there any benefits from the intervention at all?

3. Measurement of CD4 cell counts has been bypassed as a marker of disease progression. Viral loads (the amount of active virus) are more strongly predictive of illness and morbidity. Even so, is it always possible to identify surrogate markers that *fully* capture the clinically relevant end point? Or is this too strict a standard when identifying surrogate markers?

Adapted from Baruch Brody, *The Ethics of Biomedical Research: An International Perspective* (New York: Oxford University Press, 1998), pp. 180–181.

1.9

Sham Surgical Procedures

In many research studies, administration of a placebo will lead to no serious harm. For example, a study of an ointment to treat skin rashes may use both the agent under study and an ointment without medicinal properties. The placebo allows investigators to isolate the effects of the active drug more accurately, and the inert ointment does not pose a risk to the subjects. Its use is acceptable on ethical grounds because it does not pose any risks and also because subjects are usually aware that they may receive the experimental agent or the inert substance. Placebos may carry risks of their own, however, in which case their use becomes controversial.

In the late 1990s research showed that people with Parkinson's disease experienced shrinkage and disappearance of certain tissue in the brain. Parkinson's is a disease of the central nervous system that causes muscle rigidity, tremors, and balance problems. Symptoms can range from mild to very severe. Researchers were hopeful that transplantation of fetal tissue would be beneficial for people with very severe disease. The procedure would require opening the skull to transfer tissue to the desired location.

Ordinarily, researchers test new innovations for safety and efficacy against existing treatments. Because no good treatments were available for severe Parkinson's, the researchers decided to use a control group. Half the subjects would receive fetal tissue and the others would receive nothing. The researchers determined that it would be necessary to open the skull of all subjects, not just those who would receive the actual tissue, to account for the placebo effect. Patients in the control group were, therefore, taken into operating rooms and treated as if they were going to receive the tissue transfer. Some were asked, "Are you ready for the implant now?" The patients then were anesthetized and their skulls were drilled as if for actual implantation. Later, they were told that they had not in fact received the tissue.

Study Questions

1. Do you think it is acceptable for studies to have control groups that receive only placebos as long as subjects are told in advance that they might not receive the active agent?

2. Do you think it was defensible to use a placebo in this study? What risks were associated with the placebo?

Adapted from Ruth Macklin, "The Ethical Problems with Sham Surgery in Clinical Research," *New England Journal of Medicine* 1999 (341): 992–996. See also Kenneth J. Rothman, Karin B. Michels, "The Continuing Unethical Use of Placebo Controls," *New England Journal of Medicine* 1994 (331): 394–398.

Placebos and Neural Tube Defects

One reason for going forward with a clinical trial is that a new intervention might be superior to existing treatments. It becomes difficult to justify administration of a placebo instead of the experimental agent if it exposes subjects to a grievous condition. The case below raises the question of whether a trial should have been conducted with a placebo, given the possible risks to children who were untreated.

"Some years ago it was suggested that the incidence of neural tube defects in babies was higher in those born to mothers deficient in folic acid. Thus a trial was instigated randomizing women at high risk of delivering a baby with a neutral tube defect into those receiving folate supplements or a placebo. This created much controversy, as it was argued that all at-risk women should receive the potentially beneficial vitamin supplement, even if the possible hazards of the vitamins had not been assessed in case it may prevent the delivery of handicapped babies. This rather emotive argument stands up poorly to scientific logic."

Study Questions

1. The analysis suggests that there were reasons to go forward with a randomized, placebo-controlled trial of folic acid. What is the implicit rationale for defending such a trial?

2. How convincing is the statement that, in a case such as this, vitamin supplements be recommended as a matter of course to all pregnant women at risk of folic acid deficiency?

From Christobel M. Saunders, Michael Baum, Joan Houghton, "Consent, Research, and the Doctor-Patient Relationship," in Raanan Gillon, ed., *Principles of Health Care Ethics* (Chichester: John Wiley & Sons, 1994), pp. 457–469, 467.

1.11

Anonymous HIV Research

Some commentators maintain that stored blood or tissue samples may be used for research without the subjects' consent. Certainly, anonymous research guarantees subject confidentiality; however, unlike conventional research, it does not help the medical community combat the spread of disease. Participants are not individually identified or notified of results when their blood or tissue samples are tested. Therefore they do not receive potential medical benefit from tests that show they have an infection or disease.

Epidemiological studies of HIV prevalence track the spread of the virus and predict the number of future AIDS cases. Sometimes people at risk for HIV infection decline to be tested because they are worried that doing so will disrupt relationships and endanger their employment and insurability. Researchers therefore worry that enrolling only voluntary participants in epidemiological studies will not give a true picture of the prevalence of HIV infection.

Researchers at the Centers for Disease Control and Prevention designed a study that would test blood drawn and banked for other purposes. The study would "unlink" the identity of the donors from the samples and would test the blood without knowing whose it was. All identifying information associated with the samples was destroyed before testing. When conducting such tests researchers do not ordinarily request the consent of donors or notify them that their blood has been tested. Thus, no person is forced to confront unwanted and possibly harmful results.

Some critics contend that such a study is unethical precisely because researchers do not plan to notify subjects that they have an HIV infection, information they believe it is important for infected people to have. These critics also believe that researchers have an obligation to provide counseling to people they discover to be infected.

Because of concerns such as these, a Canadian medical board recommended that anonymous HIV screening occur only in concert with simultaneous public education about HIV. They also recommend an opt-out system in which individuals can request that researchers use their blood only for specific purposes and no others. This approach again raises the problem of accuracy in HIV testing: if people exclude their blood from testing, researchers cannot obtain a complete picture of how prevalent HIV infection actually is.

Study Questions

1. How important is it to have an overall estimate of the number of HIV-infected people in a given population? What can be done with this information?

2. Does the utility of this information justify testing stored blood samples for HIV infection as long as researchers cannot trace samples back to people from whom they were taken?

3. How convincing is the notion that researchers who want to carry out anonymous testing have an obligation to identify and counsel people who originally donated samples for another purpose?

Adapted from Baruch Brody, *The Ethics of Biomedical Research: An International Perspective* (New York: Oxford, 1998), pp. 70–71.

1.12

Surgical Treatment of Short Bowel Syndrome

Surgical innovation sometimes goes forward without much, if any, review by either the surgical community or an independent ethics body. Such was the case for a variety of treatments for short bowel syndrome, in which the bowel lacks sufficient surface area to absorb water and nutrition. The condition is most common in children but is also known in adults. A variety of nonsurgical therapies have been used to control this problem, but surgical interventions have been tried as well, including intestinal and multiple organ transplantations. Many of these procedures require no independent review because they are considered matters of patient management and clinical judgment rather than research.

It was only in the 1980s that surgeons began in earnest to try and transplant intestines to combat short bowel syndrome. The results of the earliest efforts were not especially encouraging, especially after failures in four children. Because of these discouraging results, one physician called for a moratorium on the procedures. Other medical centers continue to perform them despite divided opinion in the medical literature about their safety and benefit. At the present time, individual clinicians and medical centers face no barriers in performing this kind of transplantation, but they do so in the face of clinical uncertainty.

The medical literature shows that unresolved questions remain across the entire range of organ transplantation: the best treatment to control organ rejection, the best method to prevent various posttransplantation disorders, justification of using living donors for intestinal segments, high costs of both operative and postoperative treatment, and other important problems. These questions are magnified with regard to bowel transplantation. As it is, individual surgeons are free to make their own evaluations about these risks and, after consultation with the patient, perform the surgery.

Study Questions

1. Surgeons and physicians are not obliged to seek review and approval for interventions that have immediate clinical benefit for a particular patient. Informed consent remains, however, essential. What kind of information should be given to patients who face transplantation with poor success rates?

2. If the success rate of a particular transplantation technique is very low, is it ethical to offer the option to the patient and/or family at all?

3. Do you think that some instances of clinical care should be offered *only if* they are treated as formal research protocols, receiving review and approval from an independent oversight body, or would this requirement tie the hands of physicians trying to offer individual patient care?

Adapted from Joel E. Frader, Donna A. Caniano, "Research and Innovation in Surgery," in Laurence B. McCullough, James W. Jones, Baruch A. Brody, eds., *Surgical Ethics* (New York: Oxford University Press, 1988), pp. 216–241.

Trial Design: Prerandomization

Enrolling patients in clinical trials can divide a physician's interests between the role of investigator and the role of patient advocate, given certain decisions that must be made about enrollment or treatment. One way of getting around this is to pre-randomize subjects into clinical trials. Then the individual physician is not directly involved in proposing trials to patients. In a sense, the system is set up to enroll patients who have rights to opt out of the trial. While this system does an effective job in preventing bias in enrollment, certain ethical questions remain.

"Zelen in 1979 proposed a new model for a randomized clinical trial comparing a 'best' standard of treatment with an experimental one. The patient is randomized into one of the groups before being informed. The patient in the group receiving best standard therapy (G1) does not need to give informed consent. The patient in the group receiving the new treatment (G2) is given detailed information regarding the treatment and asked if he is willing to enter the trial. If the patient refuses he is transferred to G1. This method was subsequently modified, where there is no clear-cut 'best' treatment, so that after 'uninformed' randomization, both groups of patients were informed about the trial and asked to participate.

"The Zelen proposals are very useful in practice, but do present some ethical problems: patients are still being randomized into a trial without their consent, and although G1 patients are getting the best standard therapy they are unaware of possible alternatives. This may be very relevant; for example a trial of surgery versus radiotherapy [radiation therapy] where the patient may have strong feelings about which treatment he would prefer.

"Even in the modified Zelen approach where both groups of patients are fully informed after randomization, the patient may feel somewhat coerced into agreeing to continue with the trial after he has already been entered, and the investigator may feel the need to give an over-enthusiastic endorsement to the treatment to which the patient has been allocated, rather than giving a more balanced view. Perhaps, however, this enthusiastic endorsement should be viewed as part of the therapeutic strategy, thus engendering a positive attitude that appears so important in the treatment of some patients."

Study Questions

1. Why does prerandomization appear attractive as a way to enroll patients into trials?

2. In this study, patients who received the best available therapy functioned as the control group. Do you believe that it is important to advise all such patients that there might be another intervention (radiation, surgery) to treat their condition even though it is still of unknown value?

3. How convincing is the view that advising patients *after randomization* that they have enrolled in a study may coerce them into accepting their participation without further question.

From Christobel Saunders, Michael Baum, Joan Houghton, "Consent, Research, and the Doctor-Patient Relationship," in Raanon Gillon, ed., *Principles of Healthcare Ethics* (Chichester: John Wiley & Sons, 1994), pp. 457–469, 466. Text format was insignificantly modified.

Research Involving Illegal Abortions

Standards for the conduct of research differ widely around the world. The case below raises interesting questions about informed consent and confidentiality in countries that have no system to review ethical considerations. Although it is important to identify ways that the research might have been improved, it is also important to think through the standards of judgment that ought to apply to countries lacking the ethics infrastructure that exists in the United States and elsewhere.

In the early 1990s, two researchers in Argentina undertook a study of health professionals' reactions to women who enter the hospital with medical complications related to attempts at abortion. They wanted to analyze women's accounts of their experiences seeking help in these circumstances. In Argentina at the time, abortion was legal only when pregnancy was a threat to the life of the woman or involved the rape of a mentally deficient woman. Most doctors and hospital staff knew that they were required to report suspected abortion attempts, but many did not file these reports. The researchers wanted to determine whether the interactions of health professionals with these women delayed medical care, and whether the women themselves delayed seeking medical care out of worries about being reported to the police.

At the time, Argentina had no formal system for the ethical evaluation of research. The hospital had no local review committee. The researchers sought permission to do the study from the director of the gynecological ward, who advised his staff to cooperate, but no specific consent was sought from individual members of the staff. The researchers did not seek approval from the hospital because they did not want to advise administrators about the real goals of the study, as that information might put the hospital at legal risk. They also did not want to tip their hand to hospital personnel that possible delays in caring for these women were part of the study. Staff members identified women eligible to participate and directed the researchers to them. The women were asked if they would participate, but were given no clear rationale for the study because the researchers did not want to influence women's responses. The researchers did not seek signed consent, because, they said, many of the low-income women had literacy difficulties and often misinterpreted the meaning of a signed statement. Researchers did have access to the women's medical charts and discussed this information with the staff.

Part of the goal for this study was to lower maternal death rates that researchers believed were connected to worry about the law on the part of both pregnant women and health professionals. In fact, they did find that women expressed fear about being identified as involved in illegal activity. In addition, health professionals sometimes delayed providing care because of worry about the attempted illegal abortion. In talking about their results, the researchers said, "We feel that advocacy groups, composed mainly of women, can make good use of these results in trying to influence public opinion and changing the policy environment [for abortion]."

Study Questions

1. To what extent was deception involved in the design and implementation of this study? How justified do you think each instance of deception is? Could the administrators of the hospital have been told of the actual purpose of the study without influencing the results? Could the medical personnel have been told?

2. Was the confidentiality of these women well protected?

3. How might this study have been conducted so that both informed consent and confidentiality would be improved?

Adapted from Jorge Balán, Silvina Ramos, "Research on Induced Abortion in Argentina: Avoiding Self-Incrimination," in Nancy M.P. King, Gail E. Henderson, Jane Stein, eds., *Beyond Regulation: Ethics in Human Subject Research* (Chapel Hill: University of North Carolina Press, 1999), pp. 140–146.

Interim Review of Research

Research subjects usually learn about the results of a study after the study is concluded, if they ever do. However, researchers typically evaluate results at several points during the study. This is done for a variety of reasons, including monitoring for the safety of the intervention. That researchers conduct these reviews has raised the question of whether subjects should also have access to preliminary results.

Large clinical studies do not wait until all their data are collected before they analyze the results. Researchers conduct interim reviews at various points in the study. Sometimes this task is entrusted to panels known as data safety monitoring boards that, because they are independent, are unlikely to have conflicts of interest. These advisory boards are not required by federal regulation. Federal regulations require only that researchers conduct monitoring in a way that will ensure the safety of subjects.

These boards have the power to recommend continuing or stopping the study. They can recommend stopping the trial if it is too risky, or if one intervention turns out to be clearly superior to the other. In one instance, a review board recommended stopping a study when the data showed that AZT was clearly effective in reducing the likelihood that an HIV-infected mother would transmit the virus to her child. In all reviews, boards must pay close attention to statistical evaluations of results. It is important not to mistake fluctuations in data as definitive results.

As interim data come in, how should these boards—and all researchers—decide to continue with a study? Baruch Brody recommended this approach: "It is permissible to continue a trial, given the evidence now available from both the interim data and from other trials, only if it would have been ethical to commence the trial given that data."

Study Questions

1. Do you believe that independent data safety and monitoring boards should be required as a matter of federal regulation for all clinical studies that carry significant risk? Why or why not?

2. Baruch Brody maintained that studies are justified in going forward as long as there is equipoise; namely, uncertainty about which intervention under study is superior. Do you believe this is an acceptable standard?

3. Researchers routinely evaluate data several times during a study. Is there a convincing argument that these data should be made available, tentative as they may be, to study subjects as well?

Adapted from Baruch Brody, *The Ethics of Biomedical Research: An International Perspective* (New York: Oxford, 1998), pp. 156–158, 175.

1.16

Suing the Institutional Review Board

In the late 1990s and the early 2000s, the NIH, which at that time oversaw IRBs, temporarily suspended the right of a number of universities around the nation to conduct research with humans because those universities had deviated from regulations in significant ways. After modifying their practices, the universities resumed human research. In the aftermath of one suspension, however, subjects in a trial sued the sponsoring university, saying their rights had been violated. Commentators immediately picked up the question of whether such a lawsuit would threaten the function of IRBs, opening up the question of whether these boards and their individual members should or should not be protected from lawsuits.

In January 2001 participants who had been involved in a cancer treatment trial filed suit against individual members of the IRB at the University of Oklahoma Health Sciences Center in Tulsa, alleging that their constitutional right to be treated with dignity had been violated. The suit further alleged that the IRB had failed to ensure that subjects were accurately advised about the risks and benefits of the study. In June 2000 the Office for Human Research Protection found that the university IRB had failed to conduct "meaningful and substantive continuing review" of trials under its jurisdiction. The lawsuit was brought against the board shortly afterward. This suit against individual members of an IRB is unusual. It prompted worry that IRBs would be less able to recruit members.

Robert J. Levine, editor emeritus of *I.R.B.: A Review of Human Subjects Research,* said that he is not aware of any successful lawsuit against an IRB member. Leonard Glantz of Boston University said that suing a broad range of people is standard fare for plaintiff's attorneys. "It's a strategy that causes more people to be upset and, therefore, encourages institutions to settle quicker." In other words, suing the IRB is a tactic rather than a goal in itself.

Others see more lasting implications from this suit. David Korn, a physician and senior vice president for biomedical and health sciences research at the Association of American Medical Colleges, said members of IRBs "don't want to have their judgments challenged in lawsuits that charge them with reckless behavior and impose stiff penalties." Gary Chadwick, MPH, PharmD, executive director of the Research Subjects Review Board at the University of Rochester in New York, said, "Why would I even want to risk the chance of being named in a lawsuit? With the amount of research being done at major universities and academic medical centers, there will be people who had adverse events and there will be people who die. If the default is as soon as that happens the IRB gets sued, there will be no more IRBs, and there will be no more research because you can't do research without IRBs."

Study Questions

1. How significant are worries that fear of lawsuits will keep IRBs from attracting volunteers to serve as members? Do you think that IRBs should be exempt from lawsuits?

2. Should IRBs review studies twice a year, four times a year, more frequently if a high degree of risk is involved? What standard should be used to guide how often an IRB reviews a study?

3. Is it fair to expect that all IRBs function with the same degree of proficiency? Some have only five volunteer members, others have twenty members, several of whom may be compensated. Is it realistic that they should all operate with the same degree of skill and commitment? Should the law hold some IRBs more responsible than others?

Adapted from Vida Foubister, *American Medical News*, February 26, 2000.

1.17

Journalism as Research

Are the methods and goals of journalism so different from those of other areas of investigation that they should proceed without the review and approval of an independent body? The following case involves minors, their sexual identities and behaviors, and information withheld from parents. It also involves potentially illegal behavior. An academic researcher who tried to use federal money to study this topic would have had to pass a number of ethical hurdles. It is important to examine the way in which the First Amendment establishing freedom of the press exempts journalists from standards that govern academic researchers.

In 2000, Jennifer Egan, a reporter for the *New York Times*, posted a notice in an online chat room that she was writing an article about gay and lesbian teenagers and the Internet. She received a number of responses, and by meeting and talking with the adolescents, she learned that the Internet was instrumental to many of them with questions about their sexual identity. Kids who were worried about their homosexual interests were finding support from others in similar situations. Many were finding consolation in discovering they were "not the only one." Some were developing mutual interests and even falling in love.

Adolescent lust made its presence felt in these interviews as well. One young man reported that he had been visiting pornography sites and thrilling to the experience since age eleven. Egan asked these teens about sexual experiences ("cybering") that they had had online. Masturbation to sexy pictures and messages was common. Some teens had been in contact with people many years their senior who were interested in them sexually. One boy had hacked his way into the account of another boy he was interested in; once in the account he viewed and deleted messages from a competitor for his affections. Egan even traveled to a rural town in the south and met a fifteen-year-old boy without the knowledge or consent of his parents. Indeed, many parents were unaware of their children's online activities and would have had difficulty tracking these activities even if they had wanted to.

The article stressed the importance of the Internet for early explorations of sexual identity, especially for teenagers who are isolated and worry about their parents' reaction. The Internet may even be contributing to the earlier age at which adolescents identify themselves as gay or lesbian: among boys, the drop has been from nineteen to twenty to fourteen to sixteen years; among girls, the drop has been from early twenties to fifteen to sixteen years. While identifying many of the benefits of a cyberculture protected from prying eyes, the article did make clear the dangers of sexual predators. Hiding behind a computer nickname, anybody can use popular clothes and cool talk as part of a come-on.

Study Questions

1. What ethical concerns of informed consent and confidentiality are involved in conducting studies of sexuality with children?

2. A university psychologist or sociologist who wished to conduct a study of this kind would have to put the protocol before an IRB. If you were making recommendations to university researchers, what changes would you suggest for such a study?

3. The First Amendment gives considerable freedom to journalists. Keeping this in mind, do you believe that journalists should seek review and approval for articles dealing with sensitive issues? If so, from what body or group?

Adapted from Jennifer Egan, "Lonely Gay Teen Seeking Same," *New York Times Magazine*, Dec. 10, 2000, pp. 110–117, 128–133.

1.18

Equipoise in Clinical Research

When is it ethical to start a formal evaluation of a medical drug or device? In one sense, it is appropriate any time questions remain unanswered. However, physicians face special ethical questions because of their commitment to serve the best interests of the patient, not the best interests of the medical profession or of society as a whole. It can be ethically problematic for a physician to enroll patients in a trial if certain conditions are not met. The commentary below discusses under what circumstances it is ethical to enroll patients and to ask them to continue in studies.

Physicians have an obligation to treat their patients with the best known methods and treatments. This fiduciary obligation creates ethical problems in beginning and completing formal studies of medical drugs and devices.

Equipoise refers to uncertainty about whether, for example, one drug is better than another or whether a new treatment might be better than an existing one. It is ethical to begin studies when researchers are uncertain about the value of one course of action over another. However, physicians themselves may have beliefs or hunches that one treatment *is* better than another, and it would appear unethical for them to ask patients to enroll in trials under such circumstances. In other words, physicians should not ask a patient to give up a treatment they believe to be effective. Similarly, as data emerge during the course of the study that one intervention might be better or riskier than another, physicians seem to have an obligation to advise the patient to withdraw from drugs or devices that are providing less than optimal care.

Various attempts have been made to resolve this problem of what justifies enrolling and continuing patients in clinical studies when physicians believe doing so runs counter to the needs of patients. These justifications range from leaving all decisions to the patient-subjects, to oversight by data safety and monitoring boards, to conscription of subjects into trials. Benjamin Freedman believed these responses are unsatisfactory, although physicians are justified in asking patients to enroll in trials and continue in them.

Freedman believed that the reason for clinical trials is to settle professional disagreements and uncertainties among physicians about what the best way to respond to disease or disorder. The results of a clinical trial must be strong enough to change the view of physicians as a group. That is, clinical trials must produce results that are capable of influencing the community of clinicians as a whole. Without strong data, medical practitioners will remain unclear about the best treatments. Consequently, enrollment and continuation of subjects in studies is justified when they meet the threshold of credibility required by the entire medical community.

Study Questions

1. Why is it important to expect that physicians exhibit a fiduciary responsibility toward their patients? Can asking patients to enroll in research studies sometimes undermine this responsibility?

2. Why does Freedman think it is justifiable that physicians ask their patients to participate in clinical trials?

3. Interim review may justify disrupting a study if data show that one drug or device is superior or inferior to another. What is the responsibility of physician-researchers to patients when this happens, and does interim review threaten Freedman's ideas about the justification of clinical trials?

Adapted from Benjamin Freedman, "Equipoise and the Ethics of Clinical Research," *New England Journal of Medicine* 1987 (317) 3: 141–145.

1.19

Children and Lead Dust in Their Environment

Observational studies follow people to establish general patterns and pathways of particular processes. For example, researchers may study how crowds move during riots or how people in different parts of the country differ in preference for breakfast foods. These kinds of studies do not ordinarily involve an intervention. The question that emerges in the observational study below is whether researchers should have acted to protect the children involved.

Lead poisoning is a serious condition, especially in children, that impairs cognition, stunts growth, and causes behavioral problems. At its worst, it can lead to seizures and death. Using federal and state money, researchers at the Kennedy Krieger Institute undertook a study of the effects of various mechanisms of lead abatement. Their goal was to find safe and economical ways of reducing lead in housing environments. They had considerable incentive to find less expensive ways of reducing lead in the environment because the cost of full-scale lead abatement can sometimes exceed the value of a property. Would something less costly be just as effective?

The researchers identified twenty-five homes that they divided into five test groups. Each group received a different kind of abatement, ranging from a fully comprehensive program to simpler interventions involving maintenance and repair. The researchers then encouraged and in some cases required landlords to rent these properties to families with young children. They received consent to measure lead levels in children's blood at various intervals, and studied levels in the home across that time as well.

Two children under study developed elevated lead levels in the blood. Their parents charged the researchers with negligence and stated that they were not fully informed of the risks of the study.

In their defense, the researchers claimed that they had no duty to protect these children from the dangers of environmental lead. The Court of Appeals in Maryland rejected this defense, saying that healthy children should not be enticed into living in potentially lead-tainted housing and/or research programs that foresee the likelihood that some of them will acquire dangerous levels of lead in their blood. The court found that the researchers had a duty to warn the subjects of the risks because of the nature of the relationship between researchers and subjects. The court imposed on researchers an obligation to act in the best interest of the children. The court also compared this study with objectionable research in the United States and abroad.

Study Questions

1. The Appeals Court in Maryland said, "It can be argued that the researchers intended that the children be the canaries in the mines but never clearly told the parents." Do you think that the children and families in this study were ill-used? If so, in what way?

2. In what way do researchers have a duty to protect subjects in observational studies from harm? Do you believe this is a duty researchers have at all times or only in some circumstances?

3. In what other ways might researchers have determined the value of lead abatement procedures without exposing children to harm or without putting themselves in a position of responsibility to protect the welfare of the children?

Adapted from Grimes *v.* Kennedy Krieger, Inc., No. 128, September Term, 2000 (Md. 08/16/2001).

1.20

Death in a Lung Physiology Study

In 2001 a physician enrolled subjects in a study of lung reflexes related to asthma. As part of that study he wanted to know whether hexamethonium had a protective effect against substances that induce symptoms in people with asthma. In the course of this study a volunteer died, and the federal Office of Human Research Protections investigated the death and the way in which the IRB at the Johns Hopkins University had approved this study.

Alkis Togias, MD, was the principal investigator of a study of the effect of hexamethonium on lung physiology in an attempt to understand differences in lung reflexes between people with asthma and healthy people. He exposed subjects to two different substances and measured their responses. One subject was exposed to hexamethonium and developed a cough, shortness of breath, and a certain amount of decreased lung dysfunction. Dr. Togias believed that the subject had caught a cold and did not report this incident as an adverse event of the study. Another subject died after exposure to hexamethonium. Ellen Roche, age twenty-four, an employee at the institution, also developed a cough and became progressively more ill. Her lung tissue broke down, her blood pressure fell, and her kidneys failed: she died approximately one month after the exposure.

The federal Office for Human Research Protections (OHRP) investigated and faulted both the investigator and the Johns Hopkins University IRB. That investigation found that the principal investigator and the IRB failed to uncover published literature about the toxic effects of hexamethonium, which had been used in the 1950s and 1960s to treat high blood pressure. The FDA had withdrawn it from use with humans in the 1970s and had never approved it for use by inhalation. The principal investigator had conducted a review of the literature, but his methods did not turn up toxicity reports. The IRB did not request or search by itself for safety data beyond what the principal investigator provided.

The OHRP also found that the IRB failed to review research protocols at properly convened meetings. The office noted that most protocols were not individually presented because of the way in which the IRB relied on a subcommittee process. In addition, many meetings were not properly convened in the sense that they lacked required members, and serious gaps were noted in meetings' records. In light of these findings, OHRP suspended for a time the right of the university to conduct research with humans until certain changes took place. The most important of these involved the way in which research proposals were reviewed and a system of ethics education for both IRB members and researchers.

Study Questions

1. In your estimation, was Ms. Roche's death preventable? What steps or procedures by the investigator might have altered the risks to which she was exposed?

2. At the time of Ms. Roche's death, bioethicist Arthur L. Caplan said that the overall system in the United States for protecting human subjects in research "is not sick—it is dead"; it is "an indictment of our society's failure to attend seriously to a crisis that has been building for years." In what sense did the IRB fail to protect Ms. Roche?

Adapted from Julian Savulescu, M. Sprigg, "The Hexamethonium Asthma Study and the Death of a Normal Volunteer," *Journal of Medical Ethics* 2002 (28): 3–4.

2

Informed Consent

Introduction

Both ethics and the law in the West recognize the importance of respecting self-determination or autonomy when it comes to people capable of making their own choices. From this conceptual background, a doctrine of informed consent emerged as an essential standard for research with human beings. Although it may be an accepted part of the research landscape at the present time, the pathway to this consensus has been difficult and long. Some of the history that led to recognized standards of informed consent in research are reviewed in the Introduction to this book, but it is worth repeating that it was only in the twentieth century that the doctrine emerged in a formal way. Before the contemporary era, many people were used in research not only without their knowledge but sometimes against their expressly stated wishes.

The Nuremberg trials against Nazi physicians and researchers accused of inhumane medical experimentation were a signal moment in the development of the doctrine of informed consent.[1] Very few *written* documents described standards of consent for experimental subjects before World War II. In large measure, the Nuremberg Code reflects a reaction to the ways in which people were chosen at random and killed for trivial reasons under painful and dehumanizing conditions, allegedly in the name of science. The code was primarily concerned, too, with biomedical research, as against research in education and the social sciences. Because of its origin, it is no accident that its first principle asserts, "The voluntary consent of the human subject is absolutely essential." (The Nuremberg Code is given in its entirety in appendix A.)

In the United States, in the 1970s, federal regulations and the *Belmont Report* set the standards for informed consent in research.[2] The *Belmont Report* maintains that subjects should be given the opportunity to choose whether or not to participate in research, as a matter of moral respect for persons.[3] Their decision should be guided by appropriate information, assurance of their comprehension of the information, and affirmation of the voluntary nature of their participation. Information given to subjects should include the nature of the proposed study; its purpose, risks and benefits; and alternatives to participating if the study involves medical treatment. Subjects should also be given the opportunity to ask questions. Other information may be appropriate as well; for example, who will carry out the experiment, where to turn for further information, and so on.

This amount of information can be overwhelming, and the *Belmont Report* also rightly points out the importance of ensuring that the subject understands the data presented to them. Researchers have a moral responsibility to adapt information so that it is understandable by potential research participants. It should be presented in an organized way in languages (English, Spanish, Japanese, etc.) that are understood by potential subjects. The need to ensure comprehension of the study becomes more important as the study's degree of risk increases. The *Report* even went so far as to suggest that in some cases it might be appropriate to test subjects' understanding of their own involvement before conducting research. This might be accomplished through oral or written evaluations.

Ensuring informed consent also means that no coercion or undue influence controls a person's decision making, such as threats, implied threats, use of superior position, manipulation, and inappropriate rewards or inducements. All these forces may weaken people's abilities to weigh for themselves the desirability of participating in research. It may be very difficult for the poor, for example, to say no to a risky project if they are offered valuable commodities in exchange for participating.

Consenting for Others

Some humans cannot be considered competent to make decisions about themselves in any meaningful way—newborns, children, and the comatose, among others. Strict interpretation of informed consent would mean that these people should never be research subjects if they cannot comprehend the nature of their involvement. This interpretation is rightly rejected as too stringent because failure to conduct research with such subjects would leave them at the mercy of their medical disorders. For example, research on people in persistent vegetative states will be necessary to develop treatments for persistent vegetative states. Therefore, it is generally accepted that surrogate decision makers can agree to participation of these people in research. Surrogate decision makers can be parents, family members, and others who stand in a relationship of concern to impaired subjects. Using this method of consent ensures that people unable to consent are not "orphaned" by biomedicine. This is not to say that people with degrees of mental impairment (such as psychotic disorders) or mental immaturity (children) should have no say about their involvement in research. The *Belmont Report* notes the importance of involving subjects according to their degree of capacity to consent. Researchers should respect the choices of people with mental impairments and children to the greatest extent possible. They should strive to honor the objections of such subjects unless the research would offer a therapeutic benefit that would be unavailable otherwise. Again, people with mental impairments or limitations should be involved in research only with the consent of other parties, to protect them from harm.

Federal guidelines allow for exceptions with regard to subjects who cannot consent and for whom a surrogate decision maker is not available. For example, physicians in emergency rooms may wish to study new treatments for serious head injuries or trauma to internal organs. People with these injuries, those in car accidents, for example, will not be identifiable before their random accidents. As they come into emergency rooms they may be unconscious or delirious, and may have no family members at hand to make decisions on their behalf. It is possible to conduct research on these unconsenting subjects as long as a mechanism of deferred consent is in place. For example, consent can be obtained from a family member as soon as one is identified. Or, as soon as the subject becomes conscious (if that happens), he or she can be asked to continue in the study. Obviously, it is difficult to determine what counts as consent under emergency circumstances, but these difficulties must be evaluated against the problems that would occur if no research involved people in medical emergencies.

Cultural Constraints

Putting individuals at the center of decision making can run afoul of certain cultural conventions. Some cultures do not value autonomy with the weight Western cultures do. In certain cultures husbands have the presumptive right to consent to involvement of their wives, or the social expectation might be that tribal elders consent to involvement of villagers. In the United States and elsewhere, bypassing the actual subjects would be unthinkable. Although debates surround the value of informed consent in cultures that do not value independence, it remains true that for moral and legal reasons, researchers must ask potential subjects if they wish to enroll in studies and advise them of the nature and extent of that involvement. Any exception to this procedure requires strong justification, especially in countries and cultures where autonomy is at the center of research ethics.

Therapeutic Misconception

For all the effort that goes into ensuring that subjects are informed about research participation, some fail to comprehend the nature of their involvement. For example, despite educational efforts, subjects may blur the distinction between treatment and experimental investigation: they believe they are receiving a new drug *as treatment* rather than *as research* despite information to the contrary. Others appear to overestimate the possible benefits they may receive from participating in a study, and they may underestimate risks as well. Such imprecision signals confusion between direct clinical care (treatments given in the expectation of benefit to the individual) and research (studies designed to benefit people in the future). This misapprehension has been identified in various domains of medical research and can be found across the range of human subjects. It has come to be known as therapeutic misconception, to indicate that research is understood as having a personal benefit.[4]

Researchers should take steps to reduce therapeutic misconception. For example, they might restate the purpose of the study, including its experimental nature, at various intervals and remind the subjects at each visit about risks and benefits. They might also ask subjects to reaffirm their willingness to participate in *research*, with an eye toward reminding subjects that they are involved in helping to resolve uncertainty rather than being treated. As in many matters dealing with the influence of psychology in human decision making, therapeutic misconception and ways to control it are matters that deserve further study.

Deception

Researchers might not want to tell potential subjects what they will experience in a study because that information will invalidate the results. For example, if a researcher wants to evaluate whether patients mislead their physicians about taking medications, *advance information* about the nature of the study may influence subjects to make either more or fewer misleading statements. The researcher may therefore wish to tell subjects only that the study involves "communication." Thus subjects are likely to continue their conventional behavior, which is exactly what the researcher wants to study.

The *Belmont Report* acknowledged the problem that arises when informing subjects about the true nature or scope of a study will in all likelihood invalidate the results. It allowed moral justification for limited research involving deception: "In all cases of research involving incomplete disclosure, such research is justified only if it is clear that (1) incomplete disclosure is truly necessary to accomplish the goals of the research, (2) there are no undisclosed risks to subjects that are more than minimal, and (3) there is an adequate plan for debriefing subjects, when appropriate, and for dissemination of research results to them."[5] As this statement makes clear, researchers should resort to deception only when it is truly necessary and only when risks to subjects are minimal. Researchers must also make plans to advise subjects after the fact of the real purposes of the study. Deception in this area continues to be problematic precisely because it runs contrary to the doctrine of informed consent. It is morally problematic to ask people to enter research studies that expose them to risk without advising them in advance about the nature and extent of those risks. It is an open question whether debriefing after the fact does enough to respect subjects' autonomy.

Informed Consent in Practice

There are good reasons in moral theory to seek informed consent from research subjects. What does informed consent mean in practice? What information is required? How should it be presented? Debate surrounds what is actually required of researchers and subjects. According to federal standards at the present time, informed consent should include the purpose of the research; its possible risks and possible benefits for the subject, if any; alternatives to participating; the degree of confidentiality that can be expected; what compensation might be provided, including the cost of medical injuries; and the names of persons to contact in case of questions.[6]

These requirements deserve elucidation. Scientists often have a highly technical vocabulary in which they express the nature and purpose of the study. Scientific language is precise, but it may act as a barrier to understanding on the part of subjects. By the same token, researchers run the risk of oversimplifying if they try to explain a study in nontechnical language. It is also sometimes unclear how precise to be with respect to possible risks. Should researchers mention every possible risk of a drug? If so, will potential subjects simply stop listening as the recitation goes on and make their decisions without fully appreciating the nature and extent of risks?

The way in which information is presented, or the framing effect, can be influential in determining how a person interprets information and agrees to participate in research. If the project is presented in glowing language with a great deal of emphasis on its potential benefits, the subject may agree without full consideration of the risks. Other impediments to comprehension exist: researchers rushing potential subjects to a decision, speaking in language that is difficult for the subjects to understand, and so on. These obstacles to comprehension should be taken into consideration by researchers, who should make information comprehensible to subjects.

When poorly conducted, the informed consent process may be little more than an empty ritual, a piece of paper put in front of a person for a quick signature. By the same token, consent processes that are long and overly complicated may cause people to fail to give close consideration to their involvement. For this reason it may be difficult to know what standards of disclosure should be used when enrolling subjects. A good deal more study is necessary to close the gap between the ideals of informed consent—free choices made after consideration of the relevant information—what actually happens in conversations between researchers and subjects or surrogate decision makers.

References

1. George J. Annas, Michael Grodin, eds., *The Nazi Doctors and the Nuremberg Code: Human Rights in Human Experimentation* (New York: Oxford University Press, 1995).

2. For a discussion of this history, see Robert J. Levine, *Ethics and the Regulation of Clinical Research*, 2nd ed. (New Haven, CT: Yale University Press, 1988), p. 237; Advisory Committee on Human Radiation Experiments, *Final Report of the Advisory Committee on Human Radiation Experiments* (New York: Oxford University Press, 1996).

3. National Commission for the Protection of Human Subjects of Biomedical and Behavioral Research. *The Belmont Report: Ethical Principles and Guidelines for the Protection of Human Subjects of Research*. Washington, DC: Department of Health, Education, and Welfare, 1978.

4. Paul S. Appelbaum et al., "False Hopes and Best Data: Consent to Research and the Therapeutic Misconception," *Hastings Center Report*, April 1987, 20–24.

5. *The Belmont Report*.

6. 45 C.F.R. 46 Sec. 116.

2.1

Research on People about to Die

Jack Kevorkian is a Michigan physician who is widely known for his advocacy on behalf of assisted suicide. His crusade to enable physicians to help patients die led him to inject a lethal substance into a man who died immediately. Dr. Kevorkian was imprisoned for this act, which he videotaped for broadcast. It is less well known that Dr. Kevorkian also advocates research on people about to die. He believes that these individuals can be used, with their consent, to obtain research information that could not be obtained any other way. This applies not only to those with terminal illnesses but also to planned assisted-suicides and prisoners about to be executed.

Dr. Jack Kevorkian has campaigned relentlessly in favor of physician-assisted suicide. He also advocates a number of views related to research on the dying. He says the law should permit people about to die the right to donate themselves to medical research *as living subjects* for research on their bodies just before their death. He believes this would generate important research that could not be carried out any other way.

He offers guidelines on how this should be done. Researchers should not be involved in identifying and soliciting people to enter such studies. Rather, administrative officials in the presence of a member of both legal and clerical professions should obtain consent. The request should show no evidence of coercion and should be unwavering. A legal surrogate decision maker should be able to give consent for incompetent subjects. A firm negative response should exclude the subject from any further involvement in medical experimentation. A firm positive response may be reversed at any point up to one week before the scheduled experiment date. Agreement to participate should entitle the subject to counseling from physicians, lawyers, clerics, psychologists, sociologists, and penologists.

To the extent required, anesthesia should be used to protect the subject from pain. If the subject is in distress, anesthesia must be provided immediately, and experimentation may continue only if the subject reaches stage III anesthesia. The experiment should then continue until it is completed or the subject dies. Stage III general anesthesia should be achieved before experimentation on all brain-dead, comatose, and mentally incompetent persons as well as on newborns, infants, children, and fetuses. This applies to individuals condemned to death by the state, and those who face imminent death by disease or through their own choice of suicide because of disease or disorder. Experiments may be of any kind or complexity. Results of such studies should be published only in special journals devoted to this kind of experimentation. If the subject is a prisoner sentenced to death by the state, any publication of the results of the research must carry a dedication either at the beginning or end of the report citing the full name(s) of the victim(s) of the capital crime for which the prisoner was put to death.

Study Questions

1. What is the value of being able to perform studies in living human bodies, including research that might be harmful to organs, tissues, and even the life of people involved?

2. Is the mechanism described by Dr. Kevorkian adequate in identifying and protecting the wishes of a person to participate or not participate in research?

3. Do you think it is appropriate to include the names of victims of capital crimes in research reports?

Adapted from Jack Kevorkian, *Prescription: Medicide—The Goodness of Planned Death* (Buffalo, NY: Prometheus Books, 1991).

2.2

Waived Consent in a Breast Cancer Trial

In the case below, British researchers persuaded an ethics committee that a particular trial should not involve informed consent because the information to be conveyed in that process would be hurtful to the subjects. However, a subject learned later that she had been involved in the trial without her knowledge or consent. This disclosure opens the question of whether informed consent should ever be waived and, if so, whether justifications for the waiver in this instance were convincing. The case also raises the question of how to respond to a subject whose trust in physicians has been ruptured perhaps irreparably.

"In 1980, a clinical trial was initiated by the Cancer Research Campaign Clinical Trials Centre. This was a multi-centre collaborative study looking at the use of adjuvant systemic therapy in early breast cancer. Patients would be randomized to receive conventional surgical treatment—which in 1980 did not include adjuvant therapy—or to surgery and tamoxifen. The clinicians entering the trial at King's College Hospital initially argued that informed consent should be waived to avoid causing unnecessary distress to the patient by making her aware of her exact prognosis and the uncertainty of the best treatment. The ethical committee refused to waive consent so the trial was started with each patient giving fully informed consent and receiving an explanatory leaflet.

"However, 2 months into the trial, at the behest of the nurse counselor, the trial organizers again approached the ethical committee as they felt that the additional burden on patients—who had just learnt that they had cancer, and needed a mastectomy—of having to consider whether to enter a trial, was causing undue stress and anxiety. Thus the need for consent was waived, but it was agreed that all patients would receive a full explanation of the rationale behind their treatment.

"Eighteen months later another trial was started at King's, to investigate a method of improving psychological adjustment of women to mastectomy by the intervention of a professional counselor. Informed consent was not required for this trial. Because funding for only one part-time counselor was available, it was arranged so that at fortnightly intervals patients who presented to the clinic had a 50–50 chance of meeting the nurse counselor. Additionally any patients identified by the clinician as having psychological problems were referred for counseling. This randomization of a rare resource—in this case counseling time—is commonly used to maintain the principle of justice.

"In 1982, Mrs. E.T. was referred to King's College Hospital with carcinoma of the breast. She was entered into both the above trials, receiving what with hindsight was the optimum treatment of the time—mastectomy and tamoxifen. Mrs. E.T., however, subsequently found out that her treatment, rather than being individualized to her, had been randomized as part of a clinical trial, and she had not given her consent to participate in this." She complained to the regional health authority.

Study Questions

1. Do you think that the stress of learning one has breast cancer is an adequate reason to withhold from patients the knowledge that treatment will involve them in a research protocol?

2. As it was not known whether involvement of a professional counselor would help women deal with a mastectomy, do you think that randomization of women to this counselor is defensible or not?

3. In fact, the regional health authority dismissed Mrs. E.T.'s complaint, finding that the clinical staff was not guilty of professional or ethical wrongdoing. Do you think she had good reason to complain about being involved in not one but two research protocols without her knowledge or consent?

From Christobel M. Saunders, Michael Baum, Joan Houghton, "Consent, Research, and the Doctor-Patient Relationship," in Raanan Gillon, ed., *Principles of Health Care Ethic* (Chichester: John Wiley & Sons, 1994), pp. 457–469, 464–465.

2.3

Informed Consent: Emergency Treatment

The process of obtaining informed consent can consume a great deal of time and effort. Some commentators see this amount of time as an objection to the very process, especially in emergency circumstances. The case below describes the way in which people in the throes of heart emergencies were involved in a research trial. The authors of these remarks believe that some attempt(s) to obtain consent for participation in research are not only misplaced, but can lead to deaths that would not otherwise occur.

"A more serious result of the enforced requirement to obtain fully informed consent is illustrated by the ISIS-2 trial of streptokinase and aspirin in acute myocardial infarction. In this study acutely ill patients were randomized to receive either conventional treatment or the addition of streptokinase and/or aspirin (as a result of the trial now established as clearly beneficial treatment). In the UK consent procedures were largely a matter of judgment—the doctor was required to speak to the patient as seemed humanly appropriate. However in the US doctors were required to read a 'preposterously' long document and obtain written consent for every patient 'the aim [of which] was to protect the doctor, not to protect the patient, and that if the protection of the doctor from lawyers harmed the patient then that was the price one had to pay for doing studies in the US.' Perhaps partly because of this procedure, recruitment into the US trial was slow, and the trial ended some months later than may have been possible, thus preventing the saving of thousands of lives."

Study Questions

1. This commentary praises the practice of British physicians in requesting consent, compared with the practice of United States physicians. Why is the British practice said to be superior, and what is the nature of the evidence?

2. How persuasive is the statement that thousands of people died because United States physicians sought informed consent in a particular way?

3. Research would probably all go a lot faster if physicians did not have to obtain consent from their subjects. Do you believe that the need for speed in biomedical research is a reason to curtail some informed consent procedures?

From Christobel Saunders, Michael Baum, Joan Houghton, "Consent, Research, and the Doctor-Patient Relationship," in Raanan Gillon, ed., *Principles of Healthcare Ethics* (Chichester: John Wiley & Sons, 1994), pp. 457–469, 463. End notes deleted.

Deferred Consent to Emergency Experimentation

Ethics and the law coincide in requiring consent from subjects in the conduct of research with human beings. However, in a number of circumstances consent would be impossible to obtain, including medical emergencies. Rather than refusing to do research in these circumstances, various proposals have been made to study patients while protecting them from undue risk. One of these is deferred consent.

It is generally agreed that potential subjects should have time to consider their involvement in a clinical trial. However, many people in states of acute illness are not conscious, not fully competent, or lack the time to provide informed consent. Various responses are proposed for the study of medical treatment in subjects in these acute states:

1. There can be no studies where there is no informed consent.

2. Studies are acceptable when a surrogate (such as a family member) consents, but not otherwise.

3. Studies are acceptable if the treatment is likely to be of benefit to the patient and consent is given either by the patient or the surrogate.

4. Studies are acceptable if the experimental intervention is very likely to benefit the patient and deferred consent is probable. Deferred consent is the expectation that someone after the trial will see the necessity of the intervention, approve of it, and give consent after the fact.

Baruch Brody, a professor of bioethics, analyzed one report of deferred consent. A 1990 randomized trial involved giving three doses of a calcium channel blocker or placebo to patients who became comatose after a heart attack. The first dose was given within thirty minutes of restoration of spontaneous circulation, without family consent. Each family was asked for consent before the next dose was administered eight hours later and before the final dose. The study involved 368 families, and researchers later reported widespread approval of the study. "Although concerns were often expressed about the safety of the experimental drug, few families requested detailed information regarding this or the study methodology. Even fewer understood the concepts of or need for randomization, blinding, or placebo controls. Many felt relieved that something was already being done and that their relative might get 'special' treatment. Families often expressed a desire that the active drug, not the placebo, be given."

Brody believed too much misunderstanding was evident in the families' responses to justify continuation of this study or to justify it after the fact. It appears, he said, that some families were consenting to administration of the experimental drug and not the placebo. In this instance, deferred consent was hardly meaningful and in his view was morally flawed.

Study Questions

1. Is deferred consent consistent with the view that all persons have the right to determine whether and to what extent they wish to participate as subjects in research?

2. One of the core justifications for deferred consent is that a subject, on returning to consciousness, for example, would see the necessity of the intervention and likely approve it after the fact. Using this guide, is there any way to predict which individuals would or would not consent to medical experimentation?

3. Patients and their families may have an unrealistic understanding about medical experimentation. How serious was the misunderstanding in this case, and do you agree that it undermined the ethical legitimacy of this study?

Adapted from Baruch Brody, *Ethical Issues in Drug Testing, Approval, and Pricing: The Clot-Dissolving Drugs* (New York: Oxford University Press, 1995), pp. 131–144. See also N.S. Abramson et al., "Deferred Consent: Use in Clinical Resuscitation Research," *Annals of Emergency Medicine* 1990 (19): 781–784.

Research Directives

Advanced directives are mechanisms that guide medical treatment in the event that a patient becomes unable to communicate. Federal law requires medical institutions to offer information about advance directives to patients. When they work, these directives protect against unwanted treatment and secure desired treatment. It was proposed that a parallel directive be developed to guide decisions about participation in research trials in the event a subject is unable to communicate.

When people lose their capacity to make decisions for themselves, it largely falls to surrogate decision makers to decide whether or not to allow them to participate in clinical studies. For example, a daughter may decide to enroll her eighty-seven-year-old father in a study of brain function in Alzheimer disease. There is no denying that research in this area is important and necessary. It may be, however, that this man had never made his view of research known to his daughter. She may be making decisions that, if it were possible to ascertain, he would find unacceptable. By the same token, he might have been eager to be a subject, but in the absence of this knowledge his daughter could feel some guilt for turning him into a guinea pig.

To avoid these gaps in communication, some propose developing research directives. These directives would parallel the advance directives now common in medical care. The difference is that they would specify the way in which someone did or did not want to participate in research. For example, a person might be willing to serve as a subject for studies of the disease that has ravaged his or her family but not in other studies. Documents prepared in advance could help guide family members and surrogate decision makers and ease the burden of their choices. At the very least, they would provide a way to respect values and preferences when people are no longer able to communicate them.

Study Questions

1. What value, if any, do research directives have in stipulating what sort of research participation is desirable should one lose the ability to communicate?

2. What advantages, if any, would research directives have over reliance on surrogate decision makers?

3. Would it be appropriate to respect research directives that people prepared many years—perhaps decades—before they became relevant? Why or why not?

Adapted from David N. Weisstub, Anne Moorehouse, "The Advance Directive in Research: Prospects and Pitfalls," in D. N. Weisstub, ed., *Research on Human Subjects: Ethics, Law and Social Policy* (Oxford: Pergamon, 1998), pp. 195–221.

2.6

Military Exemptions from Informed Consent

Courts have consistently held that various strategic decisions of the military are beyond review. The case below raises the question whether the military's broad power of decision making should extend to experimental drugs and vaccines administered to personnel without their knowledge or consent. As it is, military personnel may not refuse medical treatment intended to restore them to active duty or make them ready for combat. At stake in the case below is a conflict between a principled commitment to voluntary consent of subjects in human experimentation and particular strategic needs of the military.

In 1990 the Department of Defense (DOD) applied for a waiver from federal regulations requiring the informed consent of persons involved in experimental research. Specifically, the DOD wanted to test a drug and a vaccine on US military personnel deployed in Operation Desert Storm, the multinational military response that followed Iraq's invasion of Kuwait. The military wanted to administer pyridostigmine bromide 30 as potential protection in the event soldiers were subjected to nerve gas, and pentavalent botulinum toxoid vaccine in the event of a biological attack.

As part of their application for this waiver, the DOD claimed that the process of informed consent under battle conditions would be too burdensome and would elicit refusals to participate, which would work against meaningful results. Moreover, the agency noted that these drugs could not be tested in normal circumstances "because humans cannot intentionally be exposed to chemical or biological agents in order to test the effectiveness of a drug." However, this exposure might occur in battle.

The FDA granted the request, but a soldier challenged the decision in a lawsuit. He asked the courts to stop administering experimental drugs without subjects' consent. The suit pointed to the Defense Authorization Act, which prohibits use of government funds for research without the subject's informed consent.

The first court to hear the case decided that the primary purpose of the interventions was military, not scientific, and that the statutory prohibition was therefore not relevant. The appeals court hearing the case rejected this logic but let the waiver stand nevertheless. Some protested this ruling, invoking the Nuremberg Code and pointing to unknown risks associated with these interventions.

Study Questions

1. Military personnel may not refuse medical treatments intended to restore them to active service. Do you think the proposed interventions fall into this category?

2. In one sense, military personnel have their rights restricted in ways that would not be acceptable for civilians. Do you think that administration of unproved therapies is defensible for the reasons cited?

3. Is it true that the information being sought here could not be obtained in any other way than either intentionally exposing military personnel to harmful toxins or administering the treatment in anticipation of an enemy attack?

Adapted from George Annas, *Some Choice: Law, Medicine, and the Market* (New York: Oxford University Press, 1998), pp. 132–139.

2.7

Radiation Experiments

A great deal of U.S. radiation research took place from 1944 to 1977 in the form of tracer studies. People were exposed to various radioactive substances to study their effect in the body. Many of these studies had no therapeutic benefit as their goal but were intended simply to describe the effects of radiation in the human body. Although most did not, several studies involved levels of radiation that would be unacceptable today. Sometimes these exposures took place without the knowledge or consent of the subjects.

From 1944 to 1974 the U.S. government sponsored various radiation studies. Plutonium injections were given to eighteen people, zirconium injections to one person, and exposure to total-body radiation to several others. Miners were exposed to radon in the course of their work, and soldiers and non-U.S. citizens were exposed during bomb tests. In addition, radiation was intentionally released into the environment on several occasions.

The Presidential Advisory Committee on Human Radiation Experiments concluded in 1996 that much of this research had been kept secret, even from subjects, some of whom had no idea they were involved in biomedical experimentation. Deception was also used to obtain the bones of dead babies to measure the effects of radiation fallout. These covert events occurred despite the fact that radiation studies were not considered state secrets at the time, and informed consent was an emerging trend.

Not only were these studies carried out in secret, the Atomic Energy Commission (AEC) took active steps to withhold information likely to prove embarrassing to the agency. In other words, its main concerns were public relations and legal liability. The Advisory Committee noted, for example, that "in the late 1940s and early 1950s, the AEC denied to the press and citizens that it engaged in human experimentation, even though the AEC's highly visible radioisotope distribution program had been created to provide the means for, among other things, human experimentation."

The advisory committee recommended that, in accordance with the severity of exposure and deception involved, the government should deliver individual apologies, money for health care costs, and financial compensation. At the very least, subjects would receive official notification of exposure. In case the parties involved were no longer living, the apology and compensation should go to surviving family members. The committee noted that since many of these research subjects could not be identified at the present time, Congress should set aside money should their identities became known in the future.

Study Questions

1. National security is sometimes cited to justify keeping certain studies from the public. Do you believe that the radiation studies described should have been conducted in secret?

2. Many studies carried out by the AEC were tracer studies that involved *very* low exposures to radiation. Do you think it is ever justified to conduct these low-risk studies without informed consent of subjects?

3. Do you agree with the Advisory Commission that the government should apologize to all identifiable subjects of these studies and compensate at least some of them? Why or why not?

Adapted from Advisory Committee on Human Radiation Experiments, *Final Report of the Advisory Committee on Human Radiation Experiments* (New York: Oxford University Press, 1996), pp. 512–529.

2.8

Yellow Fever Experiments

Is it acceptable to ask military personnel to volunteer for studies that expose them to a considerable risk of disease and death? In 1900, a United States commission began work to identify mechanisms for dealing with yellow fever in military personnel stationed in Cuba. Large numbers of troops had contracted the disease, and many had died. The commission conducted a study of the mosquito to learn if the insect was a vector for spreading the disease. The researchers also decided to use signed consent forms with the volunteers (this is believed to be the first such use). The results proved extremely useful in controlling the disease through programs that targeted mosquitoes.

In 1900 the prevalence of yellow fever reached epidemic proportions among US army troops stationed in Cuba after the Spanish–American war. A commission appointed to study the disease focused on the likelihood that mosquitoes were passing a microscopic bacterium to their victims.

Members of the commission, including physician Jesse Lazear, volunteered to expose themselves to mosquitoes. Some of these experiments were carried out in secret because exposures of exactly this kind had been condemned elsewhere in the world. In fact, Dr. Lazear and others died after being bitten by infected mosquitoes. (Contrary to a myth that has grown up, another member of the commission, Dr. Walter Reed, did not expose himself to infected mosquitoes.)

Before recruiting more subjects, Dr. Reed drew up a form that told participants what the study was and why it was being conducted. The document mentioned that volunteers faced the risk of death, although they might die as the result of other risks as well. It is not known whether the form was required by the military or was intiated by Reed himself. Military troops were not paid for their participation, but nonmilitary volunteers were. The exact amount is uncertain, but it appears to have been several hundred dollars, perhaps more if subjects became infected.

The results of the study, confirming the role of the mosquito as an animal host of the microbe, was of enormous practical benefit. As a result, a large number of mosquito-extermination programs vastly reduced the occurrence of yellow fever.

Study Questions

1. For what reasons might it be problematic to ask for recruits for research among military personnel? Would it have been more appropriate to study the disease only with persons native to affected areas?

2. Was it appropriate to exclude military personnel from receiving monetary compensation for participating? Since these subjects faced just as serious a risk of disease and death as others, would it not have been appropriate to offer some compensation, even if the money would have gone to their estates if they died?

3. Monetary compensation for participating in this trial would have been large by any standard at that time. Do you think it is appropriate to compensate on this scale when asking volunteers to expose themselves to serious diseases? In other words, is the risk of death more than balanced in this study by the potential gain of the volunteers?

Adapted from Jonathan Moreno, *Undue Risk: Secret State Experiments on Humans* (New York: W.H. Freeman, 1999), pp. 16–21. See also Advisory Committee on Human Radiation Experiments, *Final Report of the Advisory Committee on Human Radiation Experiments* (New York: Oxford University Press, 1996), p. 53.

2.9

Exposure of Australian Soldiers to Malaria

In wartime, researchers face not only difficulties of conducting research but of doing so in a way that advances military interests. The pressing need to find ways to protect troops from disease can influence choices researchers make about selecting subjects and the consent process. A wartime mentality may even influence judgments about the need for research.

From June 1943 to April 1946, Australian researchers cooperated with a British drug company to study malaria infection and drug treatments. Similar studies were also carried out with dengue fever. The medical research unit (MRU) in Australia was eager to find an effective drug to replace quinine as a treatment for malaria, since that substance had become virtually unobtainable after the Japanese occupied Java. British and United States researchers were reluctant to use their own soldiers, so the MRU authorized studies involving approximately 850 injured soldiers recuperating in hospitals as well as Jewish refugees who had joined the Australian Army after forcible relocation from Britain. The soldiers involved were unfit for front line duty.

Subjects were exposed to malaria infections, sometimes at extraordinarily high levels calculated to be several thousands of times more severe than those that might occur in jungle warfare. Exposures were by mosquito bites or injection into the blood stream. Some subjects were also bled—up to two pints—and some were subjected to oxygen deprivation and compression chambers to study the effect of malaria and treatments in pilots at high altitudes. Many subjects developed malaria and experienced shivers, vomiting, shakes, sweats, and severe joint pain. Some were intentionally untreated for days.

These men were told that their participation was essential because Australian soldiers in the field were dropping like flies from malaria. They were told that they would be exposed to malaria, but it is unclear that much information was otherwise provided. It appears, however, that these studies occurred long after any immediate threat of high malaria casualties in Australian troops. It is also true that by 1944 researchers had identified the ability of the drug Atabrine to suppress the disease if taken regularly. In fact, some US researchers worried that the effectiveness of Atabrine would lead the Australians to shut down their study. It did not.

Study Questions

1. It does not appear that these researchers described the nature and significance of this study very well to subjects. What information should have been disclosed?

2. In what sense do you think it is justified, if at all, to ask subjects to continue to face the risks of malaria even though an effective treatment was available? How might alternative therapies to Atabrine been studied under these wartime circumstances?

3. In 1999, one of the researchers at the MRU defended the ethics of this trial. Dr. Max Swan, age 81, said: "It could be argued that we had no moral or ethical right to carry out these experiments on human beings. The answer to that is that when you are dealing with a human disease which cannot be transferred to animals, the only experimental animal available is our fellow human beings. This was recognized from the beginning and continues." Do you find this a persuasive defense of the choices made in this study?

Adapted from Gerard Ryle, Gary Hughes, "Troops and Refugees Given Malaria," "The Soldiers of Misfortune," "Sweaty Shivers," "'Applaud Men's Courage'," "Painful Service Was Rewarded with Official Indifference," *Sydney Morning Herald*, April 19, 1999.

2.10

Obedience to Authority

Researchers may deceive subjects about the nature and purpose of an experiment in order to measure an effect that would be altered if subjects knew exactly what the experiment was. In the case below, subjects were told that the purpose of a study was one thing whereas it was actually something altogether different. One way to analyze this case is to ask whether the information could have been obtained any other way and whether the results were sufficiently important to justify the deception. Even if some deception is permissible, the question of informed consent remains open if subjects can suffer psychological damage when the real purpose of the study is revealed. Opinion about the ethics of this research is strongly divided. It is certainly an important study insofar as it showed that subjects's self-reports are unreliable when it comes to behavior they regard as objectionable.

Psychologist Stanley Milgram told two groups of subjects that they would be studying the effects of punishment on learning. "Teachers," as they were called, would give out word pairs to "learners," as the other subjects were called, and would punish learners with electrical shocks if they failed to remember the pairs correctly. The teachers were seated before a shock generator, with switches moving from 15 to 450 volts in 15-volt increments. The shock would increase by one increment each time a word pair was incorrectly remembered.

The teachers could see the learners in an adjoining room where they were seated, one at a time, in a chair with their arms strapped to constrain movement, and electrodes connected to their wrists. The learners were not, in fact, connected to the shock apparatus; they were accomplices Milgram had coached to play a role. They intentionally misstated the correct word pairs and simulated responses to the shocks.

At 75 volts, the learners grunted a bit, at 120 volts they complained verbally, at 150 they demanded to be released from the experiment, and at 285 they screamed in agony. At all points, Milgram instructed teachers to ignore the responses of learners and to continue the experiment. A teacher was excused from the study only after failing to follow four verbal commands of the researcher. Most teachers did as they were told.

In fact, the purpose of the study was to examine whether teachers would continue with their assigned task even when presented with evidence of a learner's suffering. To what extent would they obey Milgram's directives in the face of another's suffering? Teachers were told of the true purpose of the study only later, by which time many of them were quite upset with themselves, having learned that they were capable of great cruelty. Some say that the subjects suffered prolonged anxiety as a result, but Milgram denied this and defended his study.

Study Questions

1. After World War II, a great deal of interest was expressed in the extent to which obedience to authority guides human behavior into conflicts with moral views. Do you think that this

study is a good way to explore conflicts between obedience to authority and moral views about not harming others? 2.

To what extent was deception essential to the design and scientific value of this study? 3.

Milgram took steps to ensure that subjects left the experiment in a state of well-being: all subjects would be told that no shocks were administered, that their behavior was entirely normal, and that tension they experienced was to be expected. Teachers were also introduced in a friendly way to learners. Do you believe that "dehoaxing" can or does justify the deceptions in this study?

Adapted from Robert J. Levine, *Ethics and Regulation of Clinical Research*, 2nd ed. (New Haven, CT: Yale University Press, 1988), pp. 217–218. See also D. Baumrin, "Nature and Definition of Informed Consent in Research Involving Deception," in the National Commission for the Protection of Research Subjects of Biomedical and Behavioral Research, *The Belmont Report—Ethical Principles and Guidelines for the Protection of Human Subjects of Research*, appendix I (Washington, DC, 1978), pp. 23.1–23; Stanley Milgram, "Behavioral Study of Obedience," *Journal of Abnormal and Social Psychology* 1963 (71): 371–378; and Stanley Milgram, "Issues in the Study of Obedience: A Reply to Baumrind," *American Psychologist* 1964 (19): 848–852.

2.11

Tearoom Trade

Researchers often want to study rituals of closed subcultures. In the 1960s, sociologist Laud Humphreys conducted a study of the interactions of men who have sex with other men in the restrooms of public parks. Restrooms where this behavior occurs were known in slang as "tearooms." Despite the fact that this study was among the very first empirical studies of homosexual behavior, it drew considerable criticism. In a second edition of his book, Humphreys acknowledged the force of the most important criticisms.

To study social interactions of men who have sex with other men, Laud Humphreys lingered in public restrooms where this behavior occurred. He wanted to assess the rules and rituals of these sexual interactions in the late 1960s, a time when almost no scientific studies of homosexual behavior had been conducted. He observed a number of public restrooms in four different parks of a metropolitan area of about two million population, in a state where sex between men was a felony at the time.

From the men he met in these restrooms, Humphreys cultivated contacts, and these few men knew the reason for his visits. For the most part, however, he simply watched the behavior of anonymous sex partners. He gained the trust of the men by making it plain that he merely wanted to watch, performing the role of lookout or "watch queen." He watched from windows or doors, preparing to signal the men if someone was approaching. With his role established, he could observe the rituals involved in these encounters.

To study the men and learn more about them—how they lived, if they were married, and so on—he wrote down 134 car license numbers and tracked many of the men to their homes with the help of police records. He was able to contact fifty of them on the pretense that they had been randomly chosen to participate in a health study. Thus he obtained information about family backgrounds, marital status (fifty-four percent were, in fact, married), number of children, health, religion, employment, politics, friendships, and so on.

Humphreys tape-recorded conversations with the few men who knew what he was doing (he called these men his "intensive dozen"), but he hid the tape-recorder from view in his car when visiting the restrooms. He protected the confidentiality of all the men by keeping a list of subjects in a safe-deposit box; subjects were identified by various descriptions Humphreys gave them. No names or other identity markers appeared on questionnaires filled out during home interviews. In publishing the study, Humphreys did not reveal the identities of any individuals. Most of the men never knew that they had been subjects of a sexual behavior study.

Study Questions

1. Do you think that the researcher's intention to publish his data in a way that does not permit identification of individual subjects is adequate to protect subjects' identity?

2. What deceptions are involved in this study, and to what extent is each of them justified, if at all?

3. In what way might the information sought by the researcher have been obtained without these deceptions?

Adapted from Laud Humphreys, *Tearoom Trade: Impersonal Sex in Public Places*, enlarged edition (Chicago: Aldine, 1975; originally published 1970).

2.12

Court-Ordered Research Participation

Sometimes, courts offer drug or sex offenders the option of participating in research as part of their sentences or as a way to avoid prison. It is important to determine conditions under which courts can direct convicted parties to experimental therapies without violating the ethical consensus that people should be entirely free to participate in research.

Some judges offer people convicted of a drug or sex crime the option of enrolling in a therapy program and may suspend either part or all of a prison sentence in exchange for participation. In some instances, courts may offer the option of a therapy that has not been proved effective.

W.D. Murphy and David C. Thomasma held that it is permissible for courts to direct convicted parties to experimental therapies under certain conditions. (1) The court directive must not be coercive in the sense of being an order. (2) The court must offer a number of options, including alternatives to the treatment program that is not validated. (3) The subject's right to withdraw from the experimental treatment must be protected. Moreover, withdrawal from nonvalidated therapy should not result in immediate imprisonment but include another option such as transferring to another therapy program. (4) A prisoner advocate should be available to the convicted party.

Study Questions

1. Do you think it is a legitimate function of the courts to offer medical or psychological treatment in lieu of punishment? Why or why not?

2. Do you think it is ethically defensible to ask convicted persons to enter into research trials with the understanding that doing so will reduce their sentences or lighten their punishment in other ways?

3. Murphy and Thomasma outlined circumstances in which they think courts can offer unproved therapies. Do you think their approach adequately protects the autonomy of convicted persons?

Adapted from W. D. Murphy, David C. Thomasma, "The Ethics of Research on Court-Ordered Evaluation and Therapy for Exhibitionism," *IRB* 1981 (3): 1–4. See also Robert J. Levine, *Ethics and Regulation of Clinical Research*, 2nd ed. (New Haven, CT: Yale University Press, 1988), p. 280.

Reanimated Organs for Transplantation

The need for transplantable organs and tissues grows despite efforts to increase do-nations. The commentary below suggests that the shortage could be alleviated by using organs that would not have been acceptable in the past. Specifically, it is recom-mended that organs be taken from cadavers whose hearts have stopped beating. This practice is contrary to standards in which most organs are taken from persons whose hearts are beating but who are brain-dead. Some researchers believe that organs from donors whose hearts have stopped are not suitable for transplantation. Others believe that not only is this feasible but that use of non-heart-beating donors would eliminate many ethical problems associated with transplantation medicine. Even if that is true, certain ethical questions remain.

In 1997 a team of researchers reported successful reanimation of hearts taken from lambs and baboons that had no heart function and lacked pulse. This success was unusual because of the prevailing view that organs taken after stoppage of the heart are not useful for transplantation as they have problems that interfere with normal functioning. These researchers claimed that their techniques would be appropriate for humans, noting success in using reanimated kidneys in human transplantation.

In addition to purely technical considerations—whether tissues could be preserved and reanimated—the researchers maintained that their technique would be morally superior to practices in which organs are taken from brain-dead people whose hearts continue to beat. Family members are often asked for permission to retrieve organs from people who, although technically dead as a matter of consensus, look very much alive. If organs are taken after the heart stops, the psychological burden on family members can be eased. Using techniques of reanimation would also put an end to rumors that organs are sometimes removed from people before they are truly dead.

Reanimation would also help end the worry that medical treatment may be with-held from some people because their organs are wanted for transplantation. More-over, the technique has a cross-cultural value. In Japan and Denmark, a circulatory standard of death is used instead of the more common brain death. Reanimation would not force cultures to violate their own views of death in order to harvest organs, because circulatory function would in fact have ended before retrieval. In short, these researchers believe that retrieval from cadaver donors should be the way that organs should be harvested in the future, and therefore it should be given appropriate research priority.

Study Questions

1. Do you think that it is important to have an alternative to harvesting organs from brain-dead people, who look alive but who lack the necessary brain function to support life?

2. Do you think that reanimation of organs after heart death of human sources would necessarily put an end to speculation that treatment is withheld from people because their organs are wanted or that people have their organs taken from them while still alive? Why do you think these speculations persist, and how, if at all, would use of reanimated organs help put an end to them?

3. Based on your evaluation, what priority do you think the study of reanimated organs should have?

Adapted from Robert D. Orr, Steven R. Gundy, Leonard L. Bailey, "Re-animation: Overcoming Objections and Obstacles to Organ Retrieval from Non-heart Beating, Cadaver Donors," *Journal of Medical Ethics* 1997 (23): 7–11.

Marketing Research

The study of a drug may serve a variety of purposes, including manufacturers' interests in knowing about its marketability in particular regions. The hypothetical case below raises questions about using medical data for commercial purposes, even if there is no breach of confidentiality with regard to individual patients.

Aristide Breton is a pharmacist who works for a health insurance company as director of pharmacy benefits, which means he decides which drugs his company will pay for subscribers to take. From time to time pharmaceutical manufacturers approach him to request information about the use of their drugs. For example, they ask for the number of patients who receive a particular agent, as well as its total prescriptions by physicians covered in the insurance plan. This information can be broken down by geographic regions covered by the plan. It is possible to screen out information about specific patients, so that the pharmaceutical company could not trace the use of a drug to a particular individual or its prescription to a particular physician.

Breton is confident that such information could be turned over to the pharmaceutical company without breaching anyone's confidentiality. He suspects, however, that while the request for information is framed in terms of research about the drug itself, the pharmaceutical company really wants to study the extent to which agent is prescribed in particular regions. Armed with this information, they could focus marketing strategies on areas where the drug was prescribed less frequently than competing drugs, as well as on physician groups in those areas.

Breton wonders whether he should supply information he believes will be used this way. After all, attempts to sell the drug would proceed without consideration of whether it was the best one for a particular patient. Sometimes, pharmaceutical companies seemed interested in bolstering sales independent of clinical considerations.

Study Questions

1. To what extent should the pharmacist involve himself with the drug manufacturer? After all, isn't it true that pharmaceutical companies could review their own sales records and have a general idea of how their drug is prescribed in specific geographical regions?

2. What are the risks, if any, to patients whose drug use is being tracked?

3. Dr. Breton worries about certain risks to clinical care. What are these risks and how justified are they?

Adapted from Robert M. Veatch, Amy Haddad, *Case Studies in Pharmacy Ethics* (New York: Oxford University Press, 1999), pp. 224–225.

2.15

Pasteur's Rabies Experiments

How should contemporary analysis judge the ethics of experiments that took place long ago? Research in the past often failed to meet contemporary sensibilities and standards. It does not always seem fair, though, to judge past researchers by standards that emerged later and only in response to particular historical circumstances. By the same token, it is equally problematic to say that contemporary morality has nothing to say about the past. The following case tries to show that one way to solve the problem is to hold researchers to identifiable standards of the time.

In 1885, Louis Pasteur directed the injection of nine-year-old Joseph Meister with his rabies vaccine in hope of preventing development of symptoms after a bite by an infected animal. Although rabies was not widespread in France at that time, it was highly fatal and much feared.

At that time, there was very little ethical sensitivity to informed consent and confidentiality, but the issues were not unknown. To judge from a contemporary critic, Pasteur did little to obtain informed consent from his subjects, many of whom were children. It must be admitted, however, that parents and others sought him out and begged for treatment. In the course of his reports, Pasteur also freely published the names, addresses, personal circumstances, and treatment outcomes of his subjects.

Pasteur faced criticism about his experiments. First of all, he was accused of practicing medicine without a license. In fact, however, he employed physicians to administer the injections and did not do them himself. He was condemned for using animals for his rabies research. Pasteur, who was trained as a chemist, was mindful of this criticism, but he was also convinced that it was moral to use animals for the benefit of humankind. Critics also wondered whether the viruses he was creating in the laboratory would inflict serious damage on the entire population.

The most serious accusation, however, was that Pasteur had not followed scientific method adequately before injecting his vaccine into human beings. For example, he kept a good deal of information secret from other investigators. He defended this practice by pointing to the need for quality control: if others copied his methods, they would not do so well enough to ensure success. Eventually, he did disclose his methods to a small group of scientists and physicians. Pasteur was criticized for offering no theoretical account of his intervention. He admitted that he had not isolated the microbe responsible for rabies. If this was so, it was unclear how he could offer a "vaccine" for rabies. Critics also accused Pasteur of lying about his experiments. They said he had not conducted sufficient animal studies and was vague about what he had in fact done. In fact, his own later reports seem to confirm that he had carried out key experiments with dogs only after he had begun to treat Meister.

Most important, it was alleged that Pasteur had turned people away in the past when they pleaded for help. It was unclear why the case of Meister was any more pressing than others. In making his decision to treat Meister, it seems Pasteur violated the standards he set forth for scientific and ethical practice; however, the eventual success of his work diminished concern about these lapses.

Study Questions

1. Even at a time when ethical standards in research were not as well established as they are today, Pasteur recognized some standards that should be observed. What are the most serious ethical concerns raised about the way he conducted his rabies experiments?

2. A degree of risk will always attach to the first human subjects of a vaccine and other biomedical interventions. How might have Pasteur done more to minimize these risks to his first human subjects?

3. Pasteur's critics raised a concern about subject selection. In a setting in which many parents are worried about rabies, how do you think subjects could have been selected in a more ethically sensitive fashion?

Adapted from Gerald L. Geison, "Pasteur's Work on Rabies: Reexamining the Ethical Issues," *Hastings Center Report* 1978 (8): 26–33.

2.16

Community Consent

Bioethics analysis often turns around three key concepts: autonomy, beneficence, and social justice. This approach has seen its fair share of criticism on a number of accounts. One critic found that these core concepts were not satisfactory when trying to identify and protect the interests of communities when evaluating the ethics of research. For this reason he recommended that researchers adopt "community consent" as a fourth cornerstone of ethical research.

The *Belmont Report* is a foundational document in research ethics. It identified three core concepts important to the conduct of research: autonomy, beneficence, and justice. Autonomy translates into a respect for the research subject, especially with regard to informed consent. Beneficence deals with evaluating benefits and risks, so as to ensure the protection of the subject. Justice refers to equity in access and in the social distribution of risks and benefits of research.

Although bioethicist and physician Charles Weijer considered these core concepts to be important, he believed they do not capture another important aspect of research ethics: protecting the interests of communities. The existing framework of ethics, however, emphasizes individual rights and protections almost to the exclusion of community interests. This is especially true in societies that place community values ahead of those of the individual. Weijer therefore proposed adoption of respect for communities as a cornerstone of research ethics.

According to Weijer, adoption of this core concept would make clear that researchers recognize the status and value of communities and that communities have moral interests that must be taken seriously even if they are different from those of individuals. For example, individuals may participate in research studies such as genetic studies of disease only to have their larger community stigmatized as disease bearing. Communities can become discriminated against if their disease traits are identified and publicized through research participation of a few individuals.

It is, of course, not always clear what a community is. Communities may be defined by political views, cultural practices, ethnic identification, and even disease states. For this reason, Weijer believed that one of the first tasks of bioethics is to develop guidelines for research on different kinds of communities. That would require studying the kinds of communities that exist and their moral interests.

Study Questions

1. In what sense is it true that communities have moral interests that should be protected as researchers plan and carry out studies?
2. How can communities be harmed through research projects? Give examples of how communities can or cannot be harmed.

3. If communities are to be protected, how might they give consent to research projects? Who is in a position to identify and speak on behalf of the community? Is community consent—understood as consent from the community as a whole—possible or desirable?

Charles Weijer, "Protecting Communities in Research: Philosophical and Pragmatic Challenges," *Cambridge Quarterly of Healthcare Ethics* 1999 (8): 501–513.

2.17

Community Advisory Boards

It is one thing for researchers to identify projects they want to undertake. It is another thing to gain the trust of the people who are to be subjects; it is yet another thing to consider whether the study will benefit the people studied. Community advisory boards are one mechanism for opening communication between researchers and subjects. They can be useful in terms of subject recruitment, and they are symbolically important in establishing equality between researchers and subjects. This outreach on the part of researchers does not mean, however, that advisory boards are without ethical concerns.

In the early 1990s, researchers undertook a study on the efficacy of an HIV vaccine in Durham County, North Carolina. Research with African-Americans in that community was problematic for a number of reasons. First, there was a legacy of suspicion toward biomedical researchers. Some African-Americans viewed research in light of the infamous Tuskegee syphilis studies in which black men were evaluated but were not treated when treatment became available. Some also believed that the US Public Health Service, which sponsored the study, intentionally infected those subjects. Now, many African-Americans worried that the AIDS epidemic might be a genocidal project of the government, especially since the disease disproportionately affects blacks.

To overcome these difficulties, the researchers set up a community advisory board (CAB). The board initially had fourteen members, including an attorney, a minister, a substance abuse counselor, an HIV-infected member, several community activists, directors of various community agencies, and so on. It held monthly meetings, and members received a small stipend and free lunch. The board counseled researchers to cancel a planned survey that would have drawn attention to the Tuskegee studies. They worried that the study might ignite community concern at a critical time just as the researchers would be starting their vaccine project. The CAB did encourage researchers to represent the community in a positive light; for example, instead of drawing constant attention to its deficits, researchers could talk about the strengths of the African-American community in resisting HIV infection.

Areas of concern did arise for the CAB. Some members found themselves perceived by the community as having an HIV infection, and the board had to consider how service on the committee might otherwise put members at a disadvantage. At a community meeting, one member answered a question about whether the board could veto a question the researchers wanted to ask. The member said that close involvement between researchers and CAB would make that very unlikely.

Study Questions

1. The CAB is a kind of consultation liaison with groups of subjects researchers wish to study. What are the ethical reasons for putting a CAB in place?

2. Suppose members of the CAB wished to veto certain parts of proposed research, and suppose the researchers found those elements of the study essential to their purposes. How could this impasse be resolved in a way that is respectful to both parties?

3. Setting up advisory boards in certain communities may be burdensome because they represent one more drain on limited resources. How important do you think this concern is relative to the overall functions of CABs?

Adapted from Lynn Blanchard, "Community Assessment and Perceptions for HIV Vaccine Efficacy Trials," in Nancy M. P. King, Gail Henderson, Jane Stein, eds., *Beyond Regulations: Ethics in Human Subject Research* (Chapel Hill: University of North Carolina Press, 1999), pp. 85–93.

2.18

Subjects with Psychiatric Disorders

No person should agree to participate in a study unless he or she has an idea of the nature and significance of the study, including its potential risks and benefits. Many people, however, lack mental capacities that enable them to understand these features of a research project, whether their participation is consonant with their values, or whether the research poses unacceptable risks. It is important to study exactly the people who lack these powers to identify therapies that can help them.

In 1998 the National Bioethics Advisory Commission identified four kinds of incapacities that undercut a person's ability to consent meaningfully to participation in research.

People suffer from fluctuating incapacity that occurs in, for example, depression and bipolar states. At times they can sort through their circumstances, and at other times they cannot. People also suffer from prospective incapacities, such as occur in Alzheimer disease. They may understand their circumstances now, but lose this ability over time. People also have limitations, such as situational or localized mental incapacities. Finally, they may experience severe incapacities such as advanced Alzheimer disease or severe dementia, in which they lose meaningful sense of their circumstances or consequences of their behavior. Certainly, it is desirable to involve such people in research to find ways to manage their disorders and, if possible, prevent them.

As part of its recommendations, not acted on by any federal body, the commission stated, "For research protocols that present greater than minimal risk, an IRB should require that an independent, qualified professional assess the potential subject's capacity to consent. The protocol should describe who will conduct the assessment and the nature of the assessment. An IRB should permit investigators to use less formal procedures to assess potential subject's capacity if there are good reasons for doing so."

Study Questions

1. What are the benefits and disadvantages of a requirement that researchers use independent consultants to assess the competency of each potential subject if the subject has evidence of a psychiatric disorder?

2. The recommendation from the commission allows research to go forward without this independent consultation "if there are good reasons for doing so." Why would the commission allow such an exception? Do you think the exception protects researchers from unnecessary work? Do you think that this exception opens subjects in any way to exploitation?

Adapted from National Bioethics Advisory Commission, *Research Involving Persons with Mental Disorders that May Affect Decisionmaking Capacity*, Washington, DC, 1998.

Disclosure of IRB Review and Approval

Ethical review of biomedical and behavioral research with human subjects is a complex process governed by federal and institutional guidelines. For all the effort that goes into this review, it may be unclear to subjects exactly what it means. The commentary below suggests what ought to be disclosed to potential subjects, although disclosure may prove more confusing than enlightening.

In the United Kingdom, the United States, and elsewhere, ethics committees are charged to review and approve research proposals involving human subjects before that research can go forward. However, the process can be invisible to subjects, or subjects can misapprehend what it means.

Gerry Kent conducted a study of researchers, ethics committee members, and patients who might be asked to serve in research trials to learn what they thought was the function of the ethics review. The study showed similarities and differences in each group's perception of local research ethics committees, as British IRBs are called.

All agreed that the role and functions of ethics committees were significant. Patients especially underscored the importance of protecting participant rights. In contrast, members of ethics committees were more likely than researchers to agree that the primary function of the committees was to monitor and comment on the quality of research. Patients tended to place the most emphasis on the responsibility to avoid harm to subjects. Committee members were likely to emphasize preservation of subject autonomy.

"Currently there are no guidelines concerning the insertion of notice of LREC [local research ethics committee] approval on information sheets. On the one hand, such information is helpful and appropriate only if patients understand the process and its implications. It is possible, based on these findings, that patients sometimes expect that notice of approval implies that no harm will come to them as a result of volunteering for the study. This is not necessarily how members of LRECs view the meaning of approval. Insofar as notice of approval could be misleading, it ought to be accompanied by a description of what it does and does not imply."

Study Questions

1. Do you think the informed consent process should disclose to potential subjects that the research has been reviewed and approved by an ethics committee or IRB?

2. What are potential misinterpretations of such disclosure, and are they significant enough to withhold information that an ethics committee or IRB has in fact reviewed a study?

3. In what way, if any, is it desirable to include a description of the ethics committee or IRB role and responsibility when trying to enroll subjects into research?

Adapted from Gerry Kent, "The Views of Members of Local Research Ethics Committees, Researchers, and Members of the Public towards the Roles and Functions of LRECs," *Journal of Medical Ethics* 1997 (23): 186–190.

3

Selection of Subjects

Introduction

The way in which researchers choose subjects for studies has raised some of the most troubling ethical issues in research. In the name of science, researchers have conscripted the poor, the elderly, the mentally impaired, the imprisoned, and exposed them to harms that are terrible to contemplate. History is littered with examples of their subjecting people to painful, injurious, life-endangering, and even murderous research simply because those people were too weak to resist. As a way of controlling these abuses, regulations require consent from research participants. These regulations also counsel the distribution of risks and benefits over groups of people, so that no one group faces undue gain or loss. This counsel has not always prevailed in the selection of subjects, sometimes to tragic effect.

During World War II, Japanese researchers tried to improve their military weapons by testing biological agents on Chinese civilians chosen at random in occupied Manuchuria.[1] In some instances, they handed out candy to children: the candy was laced with anthrax. In other instances, they assigned men to undergo vivisection. Some Chinese were killed outright to study how they died. Others were exposed to bioweapons the Japanese were investigating. On the other side of the globe, Nazi researchers used humans to study exposure to extreme cold and extreme heat.[2] They also conducted genetics experiments, surgery, and studies of infectious disease.[3] Some researchers, Josef Mengele in particular, were fascinated by twins and injected them with chemicals of all kinds.[4] They also conducted experiments to "cure" homosexuals by involuntary hormone injections.[5] When asked to give an account of these experiments, Nazi defense lawyers argued that they had violated no existing standard and noted that others were conducting comparable experiments, including researchers in the United States.

The United States has certainly not been blameless in choosing vulnerable subjects for problematic research. Orphans and prisoners were often easy to enroll and were exposed to many diseases and disorders. One historian called Holmesburg Prison one of the largest nontherapeutic human research factories in United States history. University of Pennsylvania researchers offered Holmesburg prisoners small sums of money in exchange for participation in a study of personal care products such as shampoo, eye drops, foot powders, and so on, some of which caused a good deal of pain and left significant scars.[6] Many infamous examples of United States researchers using inappropriate subjects serve as cases in this chapter.

In response to public attention to research abuses in the United States, the *Belmont Report* concluded that selection of subjects should "be scrutinized in order to determine whether some classes (*e.g.*, welfare patients, particular racial and ethnic minorities, or persons confined to institutions) are being systematically selected, simply because of their easy availability, their compromised position, or their manipulability, rather than for reasons directly related to the problem being studied."[7]

The *Report* relied on a principle of social justice to ground the moral requirement that fairness be manifest in the selection of subjects and in the distribution of risks and benefits across groups. Social justice requires that researchers not offer potentially beneficial interventions only to some subjects or select compromised subjects for risky trials. It requires researchers to take into account the ability of subjects to bear the burdens of the intervention in question.

Special Considerations for Subject Populations

Certain social groups, such as racial minorities, the economically disadvantaged, and institutionalized, are vulnerable as research subjects by virtue of their social dependency. They may be easily identifiable because of the way in which they are hospitalized, the way in which their health care is paid for, the way in which they are housed, and so on. Ethical concerns are raised about whether these people might be selected as research subjects for reasons of administrative convenience, because they are easy to manipulate as a result of their illness or socioeconomic condition, or because they are undemanding in asking about the nature and scope of the research.

Current federal regulations require specific concerns and procedures in evaluating research with populations of children, pregnant women, and prisoners. These regulations are worth summarizing to provide a sense of the way in which vulnerable populations require special consideration.

Children   Research with children is morally problematic because children lack the cognitive powers that enable them to weigh risks and benefits. Although young children are not well situated to make their own decisions in these areas, it would be unwise to exclude them altogether.

Federal regulations allow research with children as long as it does not involve greater than minimal risk and as long as parents or guardians consent and children assent as appropriate.[8] The regulations define minimal risk as "the probability and magnitude of physical or psychological harm that is normally encountered in the daily lives, or in the routine medical, dental, or psychological examination of healthy persons."[9] If the risk is greater than minimal, researchers may proceed as long as the study has potential to offer a direct benefit in terms of children's medical options and, again, as long as parents consent and children assent as appropriate.[10] Some research with children is acceptable even if it involves greater than minimal risk and offers children no direct benefit but will yield important knowledge about a certain disorder or condition. However, the risk can be only a "minor increase" over minimal and must be comparable with other experiences in the child's range of experiences. And, again, parents or guardians must consent and children must assent as appropriate.[11]

A final category of research involves risk that is greater than minimal, involves more than a minor increase over minimal, and offers no prospect of benefit to the children under study.[12] Enrolling children in such trials may be important to the study of children's health generally. It can go forward only if evaluated by a special panel of experts and approved by the Secretary of Health and Human Services. Whether these safeguards are sufficient to protect children against objectionable use in research is a matter of debate.[13] However, these main approaches may be used as a starting point for analyzing the involvement of children in particular projects.

The decision to enroll children in studies should not rest entirely with adults alone. Certainly parents or guardians are in a better position to appreciate the nature of risks, but children should not be dragged unwillingly into studies. For this reason a regulatory requirement mandates that children assent to their participation unless they are so young that this requirement would be meaningless. Whether assent is relevant depends on factors of age, maturity, and psychological state. No assent is necessary if children's mental capacity is so limited that they cannot be reasonably expected to understand their role or involvement.

Pregnant Women   The federal government allows clinical research involving pregnant women as long as the following conditions have been met: earlier studies of the intervention have been done in animals and nonpregnant women, and any risk involved to the fetus is the consequence of interventions or procedures holding out some prospect of benefit for the woman or fetus.[14] If the intervention is not expected to benefit the woman or fetus, the risk to the fetus cannot be greater than minimal, and the study must be likely to produce important biomedical knowledge that cannot be obtained in another way. In any case, risk must be minimized to the greatest extent possible. Consent must be obtained from the woman. Consent of the father is necessary if the research holds out the prospect of benefit only to the fetus and not the woman, unless the father is unavailable or incompetent. Consent of the father is not necessary if the pregnancy is the result of rape or incest. If the father is involved in consent, the foreseeable effect of the research on the fetus must be disclosed. Moreover, during the course of the study, researchers may not offer inducements to terminate a pregnancy, and they must exclude themselves from decisions about termination of pregnancies.

Prisoners   Prisoners are constrained in their choices by reason of incarceration. The regimented quality of their lives and deprived social circumstances can affect their capacity to make voluntary and uncoerced decisions. Recognition of these constraints on choice has led to various requirements with regard to the use of prisoners as research subjects.

Federal regulations require that biomedical and/or behavioral research with prisoners meet several conditions.[15] The research must not offer advantages (food, medical care, quality of living condition, wages) that are of such a magnitude that they impair prisoners' ability to weigh their value against the risks of the research. Researchers may not expect prisoners to face greater risks than would be appropriate for nonprisoner volunteers. They must use fair methods of selecting inmates, a process that should usually be insulated from influence by prison authorities or prisoners themselves and that should choose prisoners randomly unless there is a reason to do otherwise. Researchers must advise prisoners in advance that their participation will have no effect on parole decisions. Other standards of informed consent and monitoring also apply.

When these conditions are met, only certain kinds of projects may be ordinarily conducted with prisoners: research into possible causes and effects of incarceration, or the process of incarceration and its institutional structures, for example. Under certain conditions, research may also address the conditions that affect prisoners as a whole (infectious diseases, social and psychological problems, alcohol and drug use, sexual assault) and other investigations of health and well-being. This is not, again, the entire set of regulations, but these procedures and criteria indicate sensitivities to be taken into consideration when conducting research with prisoners. The main point is that prisoners should not ordinarily be enrolled as subjects unless that research works to their benefit. This doctrine represents a major break with the historical use of prisoners as research subjects in all domains of biomedical research simply because they were easy to identify and recruit.

Researchers as Experimental Subjects

One thread of history in which researchers have taken the risks of research on themselves should be noted. That is, some researchers intentionally exposed themselves to severe and life-threatening diseases. Whereas some of these exposures were innocuous enough, others were just foolhardy, and in fact, researchers died. In these ventures, a scientific spirit guided decisions to face the risks of disease: these individuals believed that they were in a better position than anyone else to observe and describe the effects of a particular exposure. In other instances, researchers wanted to draw attention to and rally social support against a particular problem.

An example of modern-day researcher self-experimentation concerns an AIDS organization that developed a project in the late 1990s.[16] These activists reasoned that it would take a long time to achieve fully effective treatments for AIDS and that, even when that happened, the treatments would not be widely available or of value to people who might be protected by a vaccine. They were concerned that vaccine research was lagging far behind treatment research. Members of this organization therefore proposed that health care professionals inject themselves with live, attenuated HIV. (Attenuation refers to the way in which a virus is stripped of its ability to produce disease while remaining capable of provoking an immune response that would fight off an actual infection.) Even though the researchers planned to use an attenuated virus, they could not guarantee complete safety. According to organizers, their request was intended to invigorate research by showing that physicians and other health care practitioners were willing to step forward as subjects and show solidarity with HIV-infected people.

Researchers are not always in a position to use themselves as subjects, however. For one thing, that might compromise objectivity in designing and conducting a trial. For another thing, researchers often lack the very condition that makes them eligible to participate—they do not have the diseases and disorders under study. Nonetheless, the call to involve physicians and other health professionals who would not ordinarily serve as study subjects does raise an interesting question about whether researchers have some *obligation* to put themselves in harm's way to advance biomedicine.

Who Goes First?

As mentioned, research with hospitalized patients, elderly subjects, prisoners, and poor people attending free clinics was attractive in the past because these groups were accessible and socially pliant. Sad to say, this often reflected the view that these individuals' lives were of less value than those of others, and that risks to them therefore mattered less. This view opens the door to invidious distinctions about lives that should and should not be protected from risks of research. In a classic commentary, Hans Jonas challenged the willingness of researchers to use compliant subjects that were ready at hand.

Jonas called on researchers themselves to be the first subjects when possible.[17] All research with human beings is problematic from a moral point of view and should not be undertaken lightly. Because of the special importance of human life, he held that the primary burden of research should fall on researchers because they are the people who best understand the nature of the project and who are therefore in the best position to give informed consent. If they are not appropriate subjects, Jonas proposed that the burden of research should fall on people otherwise best situated to bear its risks. Jonas called this approach the principle of identification, and it means that the people whose education and social standing are most like that of the researchers should be the first subjects. One should not use subjects simply because of their convenience and accessibility. On the contrary, one should approach those groups only after everyone else has been ruled out. Researchers should generally avoid subjects who are poor in knowledge and motivation, and limited in their freedom; these people should be used only with a strong justification.

This approach not only provides a critique of the way in which subjects were selected in the past, but it also identifies values that should be preserved as future researchers do their work on behalf of humanity. It is important not to let the promise of scientific benefits override concerns about protecting the weak and the vulnerable. In other words, biomedical progress is not the only social good, and researchers should involve participants in ways that are compatible with social values of equity and justice.

References

1. Sheldon Harris, *Factories of Death: Japanese Biological Warfare, 1931–1945, and the American Cover-Up*, rev. ed. (New York: Routledge, 2001).

2. George J. Annas, Michael Grodin, eds., *The Nazi Doctors and the Nuremberg Code: Human Rights in Human Experimentation* (New York: Oxford University Press, 1995). See also Robert J. Lifton, *The Nazi Doctors: Medical Killing and the Psychology of Genocide*, rev. ed. (New York: Basic Books, 2000).

3. Andrew C. Ivy, "Nazi War Crimes of a Medical Nature," *Journal of the American Medical Association* 1949 (139): 131–135.

4. Lucette Matalon Lagnado, Sheila Cohn Dekel, *Children of the Flames: Dr. Josef Mengele and the Untold Story of the Twins of Auschwitz* (New York: Penguin, 1992).

5. Richard Plant, *The Pink Triangle* (New York: Henry Holt, 1986); Heinz Heger, *The Men with the Pink Triangles: The True Life-and-Death Story of Homosexuals in the Nazi Death Camps*, rev. ed. (Boston: Alyson Press, 1994).

6. Allen M. Hornblum, *Acres of Skin: Human Experiments at Holmesburg Prison* (New York: Routledge, 1998).

7. National Commission for the Protection of Human Subjects of Biomedical and Behavioral Research, *The Belmont Report: Ethical Principles and Guidelines for the Protection of Human Subjects of Research*. Washington, DC: Department of Health, Education, and Welfare, 1978.

8. 45 C.F.R. 46.404.

9. 45 C.F.R. 46.303d.

10. 45 C.F.R. 46.404.

11. 45 C.F.R. 46.405.

12. 45 C.F.R. 46.407.

13. See Loretta M. Kopelman, Timothy F. Murphy, "Ethical Concerns in the Approval of Risky Studies with Children," unpublished manuscript.

14. 45 C.F.R. 46.204.

15. 45 C.F.R. 46.306.

16. Sue Ellen Christian, "50 Ready to Risk Own Lives to Test AIDS Vaccine," *Chicago Tribune,* Sept. 21, A1.

17. Hans Jonas, *Philosophical Essays: From Ancient Creed to Technological Man* (Englewood Cliffs, NJ: Prentice-Hall, 1974).

Hemodialysis as Experimental Medicine: The God Committee

Scholars traced the birth of contemporary bioethics to concerns about the allocation of scarce resources associated with experimental treatments. In the 1960s, the issue of access emerged with regard to a limited resource: hemodialysis units. During that time, selection committees chose patients who would receive dialysis on the basis of "social worth." This process was widely criticized for the way in which certain candidates came to be preferred over others.

In 1960, in Seattle, Washington, physician Belding Scribner invented a tubing system that could be implanted into humans. It could be connected to both veins and arteries, and it opened and closed like a spigot. It resulted in sustainable treatment for people with kidney failure. An external machine cleaned their blood as it continued to circulate through their bodies. At that time, however, dialysis was considered experimental, and insurance companies generally refused to pay for it. Hemodialysis for a hospitalized patient could cost as much as $20,000 a year, and therefore Scribner's hospital directed him not to accept more patients for in-hospital treatment. But because of the promise of this treatment, he tried to carry out dialysis on an outpatient basis.

By 1962 the hospital could still handle only seventeen patients even on an outpatient basis. Which seventeen should they treat? The hospital and the county's medical society formed an admissions and policy committee made up of a minister, lawyer, homemaker, labor leader, state government official, banker, and surgeon. The anonymous committee was charged with deciding which of many applicants should be admitted to treatment.

At first, the committee articulated standards that simply required patients to be under age forty-five and to be able to afford dialysis either through insurance or other means. Still, this left too many people in the applicant pool, so the committee adopted criteria of social worth. These criteria favored the employed, parents of dependent children, the educated, those with the potential to help others, and those with the ability to tolerate anxiety, as well as people with other traits the committee saw as socially valuable. They did not, however, meet any of the candidates personally.

This selection committee received widespread attention. The news media called it "The God Committee." Dr. Scribner was uncomfortable that his attempt to obtain more dialysis machines inevitably drew attention to the committee, and members denied that they were playing God. One said, among other things, that hemodialysis was experimental: "We are picking guinea pigs for experimental purposes, not denying life to others."

This defense did not hold up for long because it became clear that dialysis was highly effective. Nevertheless, insurance companies resisted paying for it. In 1965, Congress put two social medicine programs in place: Medicare for the elderly and

Medicaid for the indigent. These programs did not, however, cover hemodialysis. In 1972 Congress finally established federal support for anyone needing dialysis, in part because of problems associated with selection committees forced to choose among potential recipients.

Study Questions

1. How did the selection committee propose to distinguish between who would and who would not receive hemodialysis? What are the ways in which this process might be ethically problematic?

2. Is it *always* ethically problematic to try to use criteria of social worth when assigning life-saving therapies? Or could the process be ethically appropriate if the right criteria were used?

Adapted from Gregory E. Pence, *Classic Cases in Medical Ethics* (New York: McGraw-Hill, 1990), pp. 320–329, 338.

Children as Research Subjects

Ethical doctrines of informed consent were drawn up with adults in mind. However, research with children is vitally important to their health and well-being. How should one treat the issue of consent with children? Should others—parents or surrogate decision makers—give consent for children who lack cognitive powers to do so? One prominent commentator contended that children should be excluded from nontherapeutic research because they cannot consent, and it is wrong to use them as means to an end no matter how noble the goals may be.

In the 1970s, theologian Paul Ramsey of Yale University held that children should never be used in nontherapeutic research if that research involved a physical aspect. He based this interdiction on the importance of respect for persons. People should not be used in research that involved them physically without their consent. In addition, involuntary research amounts to wrongful touching, battery in effect.

He stated that children are incapable of consent, and that makes them ineligible as research subjects. He believed proxy consent, from parents, for example, could be given when research held out a possible therapeutic benefit for the child in question. But proxy consent should not be admissible for nontherapeutic research, because in that case the child would be used as a means to an end, and not respected as the primary beneficiary of an intervention.

Ramsey recognized that a great deal of research could go undone if this approach was taken, but he thought it better to err on the side of avoiding harm to children, rather than exposing children to risk. He did not rule out all nontherapeutic research with children, only that involving physical aspects. It would not be wrong, therefore, to conduct observational or educational studies. Nevertheless, because children cannot consent in a way that makes informed consent meaningful, they should not be used as subjects in nontherapeutic research, even if their parents agree.

Study Questions

1. In what sense is it true that children cannot consent to serve as subjects of research?

2. How convincing is the theory that involving children without their consent, something they cannot in any case give, amounts to a kind of battery?

3. How and to what extent might research progress be slowed if children were not used in the ways Ramsey suggested? Is it fair to use progress as a criterion for deciding whether to enroll children incapable of consent?

Adapted from Paul Ramsey, "The Enforcement of Morals: Non-therapeutic Research on Children," *Hastings Center Report* 1976 (6): 21–30. See also Robert J. Levine, *Ethics and the Regulation of Clinical Research,* 2nd ed. (New Haven, CT: Yale University Press, 1988), p. 237.

3.3
_____

The Patient-Physician Relationship in Research

People asked to participate in social science research are not necessarily ill and may ordinarily decline involvement without implications for their health. When the request to participate comes from a physician, however, patients may believe it is tied to their health care and well-being. It is extremely important, therefore, to pay close attention to the way in which ill health may lead to decisions patients might not genuinely wish to make about being enrolled in clinical experiments.

It is not uncommon for physicians to offer patients the opportunity to participate in a research trial. Such requests may be extended to patients with conditions for which no effective medical treatments are available. Often, however, research may involve testing a new treatment for conditions that do have effective therapies. In other words, the physician is offering the patient the opportunity to choose between an accepted medical therapy and an innovation of unknown value.

This offer can provoke a variety of reactions. Patients may not wish to venture into unknown territory even if the innovation might hold some benefit; for example, a new drug might have to be taken only once a day rather than four times a day. Others might want the physician to decide which option to choose. Others might suspect that the physician does not really know what is best for their medical condition and go find a new physician. Patients may choose to participate or not for reasons that are unrelated to the value of the options. It is not surprising either that patients could see themselves as guinea pigs. Even after choosing to participate, patients may continue to experience strong responses. They may regret their decisions in the extreme. If the new intervention or drug fails, this may cast severe doubt over the integrity of their decision.

One of the most enduring worries about patients as subjects in clinical trials is that patients may feel compelled to participate in case their physician might retaliate if they refuse.

Study Questions

1. How strong an influence does the health care relationship and setting have in disposing patients to accept offers of enrollment in clinical trials? Is this influence necessarily objectionable?

2. How might physicians minimize the influence attached to their roles when seeking subjects to enroll in studies?

3. Because of physicians' central role in providing health care, do you believe that requests to participate in clinical trials should be offered by a third party, perhaps a medical social worker? What benefits and disadvantages would this approach have?

Adapted from Robert J. Levine, *Ethics and Regulation of Clinical Research*, 2nd ed. (New Haven, CT: Yale University Press, 1988), pp. 46–47.

Malaria Experiments on Prisoners

Prisoners were routinely used as research subjects throughout the twentieth century. During World War II they were used to test drugs against malaria. It is important to ask about the extent to which these individuals ought to serve as subjects and whether that involvement should bear on the length of sentences. In the case below, sentences were reduced, even though the prisoners were told beforehand that this would not happen.

In its June 1945 edition, *Life* magazine lauded the subjects of malaria experiments during World War II as American heroes. These volunteers were prisoners, conscientious objectors, and hospital patients. They were knowingly infected with malaria to test Atabrine, an antimalarial drug. The prisoners were infected with malaria through mosquito bites and other means. They were then followed as they progressed through various stages of the disease. Some of them became quite sick. In addition to studying the path of disease progression, the researchers assessed the effect of drug therapies given at various points during illness.

Nathan Leopold was one of the prisoner volunteers. His incarceration for kidnap and murder cut short a promising education in law, not to mention the life of a twelve-year-old boy. Leopold viewed participating in the malaria experiments as a way of aiding the war effort and expressing his patriotism.

In his 1958 autobiography he stated that he "wanted very badly to do my bit [in the war, and] being a malaria volunteer represented by far my best opportunity . . . Here was a chance to get in a payment on my debt, an opportunity much more important and favorable than most to expiate some part of my guilt." He also wrote about why his fellow prisoners volunteered for the research. "A number of men had relatives or friends in the armed services; they were more than glad to do what they could if it would help the soldiers. Many took part because they hoped that their sentences would be reduced; some few actually took malaria to earn the hundred dollars [incentive payment]."

Leopold was emphatic that "no man was coerced or even persuaded" to be a research subject, and all volunteers were treated in a "scrupulously ethical manner." All told, there was an excess of subjects because the trial was connected with the war effort and because patriotism was high. Nevertheless, Leopold's account states that some of the subjects were motivated by their desire to leave prison.

Study Questions

1. Despite being told that their sentences would not be shortened if they volunteered as research subjects, many prisoners continued to believe that they would. In fact, the governor of Illinois did release some of these men before their sentences were completed because of their participation. Is it defensible to shorten prison sentences for this reason?

2. During World War II there was no shortage of patriotic prisoners ready to expose themselves to malaria. Do you think that prisoners' choice to volunteer for research is unaffected by their circumstances? Does imprisonment lead men to decisions they would not otherwise make?

3. If you accept the notion that prisoners may ethically participate as research subjects, is it also fair to give them money or other items of value in exchange for participation?

Adapted from Jonathon Moreno, *Undue Risk: Secret State Experiments on Humans* (New York: W.H. Freeman, 2000), pp. 32–34; Nathan Leopold, *Life Plus 99 Years* (Garden City, NJ: Doubleday, 1958).

Prisoners as Research Subjects

The enduring concern about prisoners being subjects of biomedical research is that their circumstances make it impossible for them to consent freely. Use of captive populations for research is filled with historical examples of abuse. In the case below, prisoners argued before a court that they should not be subjects because being offered the opportunity to participate was by its very nature coercive. The court held otherwise, but the autonomy of prisoners is still very much a live question.

In 1979 a group of prisoners filed a lawsuit claiming wrongful treatment as research subjects. They claimed that "poor prison conditions, idleness, and high level of pay relative to other prison jobs rendered their participation in medical studies coerced and in violation of their constitutional rights to due process, privacy, and protection against cruel and unusual punishment."

The judge rejected most of the argument. In his opinion on the matter, he wrote, "Plaintiffs have not proven any violations of their constitutional rights. . . . Some persons may prefer that if society's needs require that human beings be subjects of non-dangerous, temporarily disabling, unpleasant medical experiments, such subjects should either be chosen by lot or at least not come solely from the ranks of the socially or economically underprivileged, including prison inmates. Such preference, however, even if valid, does not add up to a presently established constitutional absolute." The judge held that there is no absolute bar to doing research with prisoners but did admit the need for serious oversight and regulation.

Study Questions

1. In what sense could the conditions of prison coerce prisoners into studies, and are these conditions strong enough to rule out ever using prisoners for research?

2. The judge found that asking prisoners to participate in research violated no aspect of the Constitution. What reasons might have led him to underline the need for oversight and regulation?

3. Should prisoners receive reduced sentences or preferential treatment because of their participation as research subjects?

Adapted from Robert J. Levine, *Ethics and Regulation of Clinical Research*, 2nd ed. (New Haven, CT: Yale University Press, 1988), p. 281.

3.6

Spouse Consent to Research Participation

One way to approach consent in countries around the world is to observe existing standards. In some cultures husbands make decisions about the activities of their wives. If researchers from the United States were to respect local customs, they would approach husbands and not wives when recruiting subjects. This approach clearly runs afoul of ethical and legal imperatives in the United States and other developed countries to secure the informed consent of subjects.

In some countries, husbands decide many of the activities their wives may engage in. This extends to participation in research studies. Researchers face dilemmas when trying to design studies involving these women. Ethical and legal requirements in many nations require consent from the person under study unless that person is incapable of making decisions. If researchers strictly observed these standards, they could not study issues important to women.

A program of the World Health Organization recognized this problem and held that it should not sponsor studies that do not respect the autonomy of subjects and their right to confidentiality. However, this program—the Scientific and Ethical Review Group of the Special Programme of Research, Development, and Research Training in Human Reproduction—does recognize the need for accommodation of cultures in which men's decisions prevail over those of women.

It states, "In rare circumstances, it may be necessary for researchers to conform to local custom and request partner agreement. An example would be the impossibility of recruiting any research subjects for a study in a particular country without partner agreement and the subsequent impossibility of gaining approval in that country for a new contraceptive drug or device. If failure to conduct the research would result in an inability of people in that country to receive the benefits of the drug or device, this consequence might be judged as sufficiently negative for the common good of the public to outweigh the usual prohibition against partner agreement for the individual subject."

Study Questions

1. In cultures that do not value a spouse's independent status and choices, how serious do you believe it is to depart from the standard that subjects should make decisions for themselves about participating in research?

2. What is the rationale given by the WHO program for accommodating, in some instances, the spouse's right to consent on behalf of his wife? Does the justification appeal to the need to observe local customs, or is there another reason? How convincing is this reason that spouses should be involved?

Adapted from Ruth Macklin, "Is Ethics Universal? Gender, Science, and Culture in Reproductive Health Research," in Nancy M. P. King, Gail E. Henderson, Jane Stein, eds., *Beyond Regulations: Ethics in Human Subjects Research* (Chapel Hill: University of North Carolina Press, 1999), pp. 23–44.

Is There a Duty to Serve as a Research Subject?

In one of the truly classic essays on biomedical ethics, German philosopher Hans Jonas outlined a view that progress in research is an optional goal and that it generally does not create duties of participation. That being the case, researchers offer their work to the public as a kind of gift. They cannot ask others to involve themselves in risk as a matter of duty. The summary of this argument below outlines a ladder of priority for choosing subjects—the principle of identification. Jonas contended that when they can, researchers should consider themselves first in line for their experiments. In many ways, this article, written in 1969, was a response to atrocities in World War II. It is well worth asking how its message bears on the design of clinical trials today.

Few diseases threaten the existence of society as a whole. Consequently, it is not accurate to say that medical research is necessary to the continued existence of society. Progress is an optional goal and therefore certain moral constraints affect ways in which research may be conducted. Participation is optional and not a duty. If disease and disorders threatened society as a whole, some degree of obligation might prevail, but for the most part society can absorb the individual tragedies that diseases cause.

It follows, then, that people who are sick should not be conscripted into studies. They are society's special trust and should not be asked to face additional risks and burdens. However, no conquest of disease would be possible if the sick were not enrolled as research subjects. Their total exemption would defeat the purpose of research.

As a matter of moral logic, it should be researchers who are involved first and foremost as subjects, because they know the risks best and because their involvement asserts identification with the sick. However, they cannot always be useful in this regard. Therefore, they should involve subjects most like themselves in terms of motivation, identification with the project, and capacity for understanding the meaning of participation. This is always going to be difficult because sickness weakens these capacities. Ironically, it is the very factors that make patients accessible for experimentation that should make us morally cautious about their involvement. Nevertheless, researchers should avoid subjects who are poor in knowledge, motivation, and freedom of decision. They should have compelling justification to enroll such subjects.

This hierarchy reverses the prevailing selection of subjects who are chosen simply because they are available. We have a sense of a sacrifice of the few for the many in terms of life and happiness, and that this sacrifice is not always voluntary. We should ask, who is to be martyred? In the service of what cause? And why?

Study Questions

1. According to this analysis, research is a gift to society and biomedical progress is an optional goal. How convincing is this view?

2. How convincing is the view that researchers should, to the extent possible, choose themselves first as subjects of their studies? Would it not be more desirable to enroll people who contribute little to society to face risks of harm, disability, and even death?

3. According to this analysis, the people least well-situated to understand and appreciate the nature of research should be recruited last, if at all, into studies. Is this approach overly protective and does it take away decisions from adults who should be respected for their own decisions?

Adapted from Hans Jonas, *Philosophical Essays: From Ancient Creed to Technological Man* (Englewood Cliffs, NJ: Prentice-Hall, 1974).

Live Cancer Cell Injections

Many interventions that researchers believe to be safe provoke concern in the public. The case below involves exactly such a study, in which live human cancer cells were injected into chronically ill, hospitalized patients. What's more, these injections were made without the knowledge or consent of the patients. This study is a landmark in research ethics, and it raises questions about the extent to which paternalism should prevail in making decisions about what subjects should be told.

In 1963 researchers from the Sloan–Kettering Institute for Cancer Research in New York approached the Jewish Chronic Disease Hospital in Brooklyn and asked them to participate in a study that entailed injecting live cancer cells under the skin of chronically ill and debilitated patients. The research team, led by Chester M. Southam, MD, explained that the goal was to measure the immune response to the challenge of foreign cells. They wanted to know how long it would take the bodies of these patients to reject the cancerous cells. They said this knowledge was important in understanding the diagnosis and treatment of cancer.

With the approval of the director of medicine at the Brooklyn hospital, three doctors injected such cells into twenty-two patients at two sites on the thigh or arm, and observed the subjects at weekly intervals for six weeks. Several blood samples were taken to measure various antibody reactions. The doctors did not inform the patients that the purpose of these injections was experimental; in fact, they did not disclose the real reason for the injections at all. It appears that the patients were told only that these were skin tests. The cancer cells grew for a time under the skin, producing small nodules that eventually disappeared without any effect on patients' overall health.

The hospital board learned of these studies, and one member, Dr. Hyman Strauss, instituted legal proceedings against the hospital in an effort to learn more about them. He went to three courts before being upheld in the right to review patient records. He claimed that one of the purposes of the study had been to see whether cancer could be induced in humans by injecting live cancer cells.

Southam, however, denied that this was even a possibility. In defending his research, he said, "It is, of course, inconsequential whether these are cancer cells or not, since they are foreign to the recipient and hence rejected. The only drawback to the use of cancer cells is the phobia and ignorance that surrounds the word 'cancer.'" He concluded that the injections were less dangerous than skin grafts would have been.

In fact, similar studies had been conducted at other sites. When asked about the issue of consent, Southam said, "You ask me if I obtained (written) permission from our patients before doing these studies. We do not do so at Memorial or James Ewing Hospital [other sites where such experiments were carried out] since we now regard it as a routine study, much less dramatic and hazardous than other routine procedures such as bone marrow aspiration and lumbar puncture. We do not get signed permits from our volunteers at the Ohio State Penitentiary but this is because of the law-oriented personalities of these men, rather than for any medical reason." Southam also noted that this research would not involve any expense for the hospital or the patients.

While insisting on the safety of the studies, Southam did spell out the reasons he did not want to be a subject himself, in spite of lack of evidence that the injections would produce cancer. "I would not have hesitated if it would have served a useful purpose," he said, but "to me it seemed like false heroism, like the old question whether the general should march behind or in front of his troops. I do not regard myself as indispensable—if I were not doing this work someone else would be— and I did not regard the experiment as dangerous. But, let's face it, there are relatively few skilled cancer researchers, and it seemed stupid to take even the little risk."

Study Questions

1. What deception, if any, occurred in this study?

2. How defensible was the selection of subjects? Even if subjects had been informed of the nature of the research, do you think that they were the most appropriate population in which to carry out the study?

3. What other ways might have been used to obtain the results of interest to the researchers?

Adapted from Jay Katz, Alexander Morgan Capron, Eleanor Swift Glass, *Experimentation with Human Beings: The Authority of the Investigator, Subject, Professions, and State in the Human Experimentation Process* (New York: Russell Sage Foundation, 1972), pp. 9–65. See also Lawrence K. Altman, *Who Goes First? The Story of Self-Experimentation in Medicine* (Berkeley: University of California Press, 1998), pp. 296–297.

Self-Experimentation: The Peruvian Medical Student Hero

The history of medicine contains signal instances in which researchers took it upon themselves to face medical risks of unknown consequences. In the following case from the late nineteenth century, a young researcher paid the ultimate price for his experiment, even as he made a signal contribution in showing that different symptoms could be manifested in the same disease.

The disorder verruga peruana causes wartlike growths on the skin and in the mouth. These are in fact tumors of blood vessels. The disease produces a debilitating fever and severe joint pain, and can be fatal. It was once common in the steep Andes valleys of Peru, Ecuador, and Colombia.

Daniel Carrión, a medical student, had been studying these symptoms and their geographic distribution. It was not known at this time, however, if the symptoms were elements of one disease or two. Carrión wanted to study the evolution of the skin bumps and decided it would be necessary to inject material from a verruga growth into a healthy person. Thus it would be possible to learn about the incubation period and whether the condition was transmissible. The disease was puzzling enough that a Peruvian medical society announced a prize for contributions to its study.

Friends and professors tried to dissuade Carrión from experimenting on himself, but he said the problem was a Peruvian one and that it should be a Peruvian who solved it. Therefore, on August 27, 1885, he lanced a verruga in a young boy, expressed some of the material, and injected it into his own arm. On September 21, he began making diary entries, noting vague discomfort and pains in his left ankle. On September 23, he had greater discomfort, with high fever and chills, vomiting, abdominal cramps, and pain in his bones and joints. He could not eat, and his thirst could not be quenched. By September 26, he was no longer able to maintain the diary, although his mind remained alert. He developed severe anemia and a heart murmur. In fact, he concluded that verruga and fever had the same origin. He was scheduled for blood transfusions that never occurred, but blood typing was at this point still unknown, and the transfusions might have been fatal in any case. On October 5, he died.

Carrión was widely eulogized, and a statue was erected to him in Lima. However, one doctor criticized the experiment as a horrible act by a naive young man that disgraced the profession. Others said he effectively committed suicide. Police filed murder charges against a physician who had assisted this "horrible act" by helping Carrión with his injections, but these charges were later dropped. Carrión is still respected for having linked diverse symptoms to a single root, something not well understood at the time.

In 1937, Max Kuczynski-Godard, a physician and bacteriologist in Peru, repeated this kind of self-experiment, injecting himself with a culture of the bacterium

Bartonella bacilliformis. He studied skin biopsies from the affected site; he also developed the disease but apparently did not die. With this contribution, there was confirmation of a common causal agent.

Study Questions

1. Could this information have been obtained without putting the researcher's life at risk?

2. Even if a researcher is willing to assume the risk of death, what mechanism or method might be used to ensure that the researcher has no ill-considered reason for exposing himself or herself to those risks?

Adapted from Lawrence K. Altman, *Who Goes First? The Story of Self-Experimentation in Medicine* (Berkeley: University of California Press, 1998), pp. 1–4.

Self-Experimentation: Cancerous Tissue

Although self-experimentation is not the dominant trend in medicine, several well-known examples exist of researchers using themselves as the first subjects of investigations. The case below surveys experiments of various researchers who put malignant tissues into their own bodies. These attempts certainly bypass the problem of informed consent in others, but they also raise questions about the ethics of subjecting oneself to unknowable risks. No adverse circumstances came out of the experiments, but it is worth examining the ethics involved.

In 1777 Dr. James Nooth, surgeon to the Duke of Kent and member of the Royal College of Surgeons, inserted cancerous tissue into a small incision in his own arm. Some inflammation and minor pain followed, but he did not develop cancer. He repeated the experiment several times.

In 1808 Dr. Jean Louis Alibert, personal physician to Louis XVIII, instructed a colleague to inject him with liquid taken from a woman who had breast cancer. This injection was later repeated. He experienced some inflammation but no cancer.

In 1901 Dr. Nicholas Senn of Chicago took a malignant lymph node from a man with lip cancer and implanted it under the skin of his own forearm. A nodule formed, followed by inflammation, but the nodule disappeared, and the only aftereffect was a small scar. Senn wanted to demonstrate his belief that cancer was neither contagious nor communicable. In defending this view, he pointed out that there was no evidence that surgeons who cut their fingers or hands during surgery to remove tumorous growths had ever developed cancer that way.

In 1954 and 1955 Dr. Thomas E. Brittingham III received injections of blood taken from a woman with myelogenous leukemia. He did this ten times: once a week for nine consecutive weeks and once more three months later. He received about a quart of blood in total. He wanted to study the transmissibility of cancer as well as the effect of white cell antibodies after multiple transfusions. For the most part, he experienced no major adverse effects, although after one injection he did have a bout of coughing, headache, nausea, back discomfort, chills, and fever. His reaction supported the view that white blood cells were responsible for some of the ill effects of blood transfusions. He did not show signs of cancer.

Brittingham then injected himself with the blood of ten other patients with various blood disorders. During these injections he experienced one serious, life-threatening setback with vomiting, diarrhea, chills, fever, dangerously low blood pressure levels, and other symptoms. He came close to death, but eventually recovered having sustained some liver damage and a minor blood clot.

In 1956 Brittingham underwent eleven other injections of normal white blood cells, and these studies sometimes involved bone marrow tests. This time he wanted to test the body's capacity to react to white blood cells despite absence of antibodies in the blood stream.

Also in 1956 he injected himself twenty-three times over an eight-month period with leukemic white cells. He became sick after most of these injections, but he wanted to know whether the injection of leukemic white cell antibodies into leukemic patients might suppress cancer by attacking the diseased cells. His blood was treated to produce a serum that was then injected into the patient who had donated the leukemic cells. The patient's white cell count dropped, which is desirable since leukemia causes uncontrolled white blood cell proliferation, but the drop was only temporary. Brittingham's work is regarded as a pioneering effort in cancer immunotherapy.

In 1960 Brittingham received more injections of blood from a seventy-year-old woman with chronic lymphocytic leukemia. Despite all of these experiments, he never developed leukemia. Although he died of cancer of the kidney in 1986, there was no reason to believe it was connected to his self-experiments.

During his lifetime and since some commentators have called Brittingham's experiments self-destructive and likened them to suicide attempts. Others said they represented heroic medical progress. In retrospect, Brittingham thought himself wrong to have overlooked his obligations to his wife and four children. After hearing such criticism, he once responded, "At the time I did not think my death would have been a disaster to my wife or children. Now that's a good example of making your thinking meet the circumstances! It wouldn't have bothered me to die then. But it would have bothered them a lot. It was awfully wrong from that standpoint, as I only came to understand later."

Study Questions

1. Is a researcher justified in assuming any amount of risk to advance scientific knowledge? How do researchers' other obligations, to family, for example, figure into an ethical assessment of risks they should accept?

2. One of the benefits of requiring that research studies be reviewed and approved in advance is that independent committees can make recommendations about the disclosure of risks and benefits. What risks do you think Dr. Brittingham faced, and how do you think these risks should be presented if the research were carried out with other subjects?

3. Do you think that, insofar as they can, physicians and other researchers ought to include themselves in their own studies?

Adapted from Lawrence K. Altman, *Who Goes First? The Story of Self-Experimentation in Medicine* (Berkeley: University of California Press, 1998), pp. 283–297.

Self-Experimentation: AIDS Vaccine

Researchers enroll themselves in clinical trials for many reasons. One is to create a sense of solidarity with those who suffer from a particular disorder. Another is to signal the safety of an intervention to the public. The case below raises questions with regard to a socially provocative disease.

In 1986 Dr. Daniel Zagury, of the Pierre-et-Marie Curie University in Paris, became the first subject of an AIDS vaccine study by injecting the vaccine into his body. Specifically, he injected a virus known to be harmless but that had been modified by inserting a protein from the outer core of HIV. The goal was to identify a modification of HIV that would provoke an immune reaction in the body, but would be harmless itself. It was hoped that the altered vaccinia virus would provoke the body's immune system into mounting a defense that would protect it in case of a real HIV infection. (Modified vaccinia virus is often used in vaccine studies as a mechanism of delivery.)

At this stage, the aim was to learn whether the altered virus could be put into human bodies safely. Because Zagury did not develop toxic reactions or symptoms of AIDS, he concluded that this signaled short-term safety of the vaccine. However, people who undergo this intervention may test positive for HIV infection for the rest of their lives even if they do not have the infection.

Zagury went on to work on an altered virus that drew a protein from the inner core of HIV. It was hypothesized that use of this protein may provide a defense against a broader array of the varieties of HIV. When such a vaccine became available, Dr. Zagury said he wanted to be among the first to take it.

Study Questions

1. What are the risks—medical and social—to people involved in a clinical trial of an AIDS vaccine, especially if that vaccine makes them appear that they are infected with HIV?

2. How might people in clinical trials be protected from social discrimination?

3. One complication of HIV vaccine trials is that subjects must be exposed to the virus in order to test the adequacy of the immune response. But researchers do not know whether or not a vaccination will, in fact, stop the infection. How should researchers handle this dilemma? They want subjects to expose themselves to HIV, but they also have an obligation to tell subjects that the vaccine may not protect them in the event of exposure to HIV.

Adapted from Lawrence K. Altman, *Who Goes First? The Story of Self-Experimentation in Medicine* (Berkeley: University of California Press, 1998), pp. 283–297.

3.12

Radiation Studies: Tracer Studies in Children

Tracer studies follow the dispersal of radioactive elements throughout the human body. From the 1940s on, the federal government sponsored a variety of these studies, some in children. For the most part, the studies did not present significant risks to subjects, although some clearly did. In the case below, it is clear that information presented to parents of institutionalized children was highly manipulated. Over and above deficits of informed consent, what lessons, if any, may be drawn from the study of historical examples of ethical lapse?

In the 1940s and 1950s no specific rules governed biomedical research with children; however, an Atomic Energy Commission subcommittee did issue guidelines for studying radioisotopes in children. In general, these guidelines discouraged use of radioisotopes in normal children, but they did allow exceptions. The Subcommittee on Human Applications could accept studies with children who were not patients if they were necessary to study an important problem that could not be assessed by other methods, and if the dose of radioactive materials was low enough to be considered harmless. For all that, these guidelines made no mention of consent, and "important" and "harmless" were not defined.

In 1946, researchers at the Massachusetts Institute of Technology exposed seventeen children to radioactive iron at the state Fernald School which cared for retarded children. A second study from 1950–1953 exposed fifty-seven subjects to radioactive calcium. Neither study had any intended therapeutic benefit for the children. They involved very low dosages of radiation, and it is unlikely that any of the children were harmed.

Several letters were sent to solicit consent from parents to these studies. A first letter made reference to a nutritional study in which children would receive a special diet rich in cereal, iron, and vitamins. Parents were told further that "it will be necessary to make some blood tests at stated intervals, similar to those to which our patients are already accustomed, and which will cause no discomfort or change in their physical condition other than possibly improvement." This letter made no mention of isotopes or risks associated with radioactivity. A second letter to solicit consent from parents is reprinted in its entirety below.

May 1953

Dear Parent:

In previous years we have done some examinations in connection with the nutritional department of the Massachusetts Institute of Technology, with the purposes of helping to improve the nutrition of our children and to help them in general more efficiently than before.

For the checking up of the children, we occasionally need to take some blood samples, which are then analyzed. The blood samples are taken after one test meal which consists of a special breakfast meal containing a certain amount of calcium. We have asked for volunteers to give a sample of blood once a month for three months, and your son has agreed to volunteer because the boys who belong to the Science Club have many additional privileges. They get a quart of milk daily during that time, and are taken to a baseball game, to the beach, and to some outside dinners and they enjoy it greatly.

I hope that you have no objection that your son is voluntarily participating in this study. The first study will start on Monday, June 8th, and if you have not expressed any objections we will assume that your son may participate.

Sincerely yours,
Clemens E. Benda, M.D.
Clinical Director

Approved:
Malcolm J. Farrell, M.D.
Superintendent

Study Questions

1. Did this consent mechanism for enrolling children adequately disclose the nature, purpose, and any risks of the study?

2. Did the consent mechanism contain objectionable inducements to have parents agree to the participation of their children?

Adapted from Advisory Committee on Human Radiation Experiments, *Final Report of the Advisory Committee on Human Radiation Experiments* (New York: Oxford University Press, 1996), pp. 203–204, 210–211.

3.13

Is Stuttering Innate or Learned?

Depending on the theory of its cause, a disorder can be treated in different ways. In the early part of the twentieth century there was a consensus that stuttering was biological in origin. As a result, various medical treatments were pursued. One researcher tried to show, however, that stuttering could be learned, that it was not biologically determined. If that were the case, various strategies should be avoided in diagnosing and treating it. To prove his point, the researcher tried to induce stuttering in normal-speaking subjects. The outcome had profound implications for the way in which therapy should be designed.

Wendell Johnson grew up a stutterer. He pursued many therapies for this difficulty: hypnotism, psychoanalysis, electric aversion therapy, and cold water therapy. He once had his dominant arm, the right, placed in a cast, on the theory that forcing him to use his left arm would equalize an imbalance of the brain that was responsible for stuttering. In fact, stuttering so preoccupied Johnson that he became a professor of speech pathology, with stuttering as a primary focus of his research. By 1936 he began to resist the prevailing theory that stuttering was due to an innate or biological cause. He believed that it was due to harsh attention being drawn to a child's normal and exploratory repetition of syllables and words. In effect, it was the diagnosis of stuttering that locked children into patterns of stuttering.

At the University of Iowa, Professor Johnson hired Mary Tudor as an assistant in a study of this theory. In January 1939, Tudor started her assignment at the Iowa Soldiers' Orphans' Home in Davenport, Iowa, which had given permission for the study. The Home housed 500 to 600 orphans and neglected children. The study screened 256 children to select 22 subjects, 10 stutterers and 12 normal speakers ranging in age from 7 to 15 years. Both stutterers and normal speakers were divided into two subgroups labeled stutterers or nonstutterers. In each group of nonstutterers, Tudor used positive encouragement to help children get past speech problems she observed. In each group labeled stutterers, she drew exaggerated and sharp attention to speech problems to heighten children's consciousness about stuttering, to the point at which anxiety produced the very effect of stuttering. At Johnson's recommendation, Tudor lied to teachers at the Home, telling them that she was there to do speech therapy. This deception helped the experiment: as she labeled children as stutterers, teachers would pick up the label and treat the children as stutterers as well.

Several children labeled as stutterers who had previously shown no signs of the problem developed stuttering patterns, including word duplication in written assignments. Students who already were afflicted showed heightened patterns of stuttering. In all, speech deteriorated for five of the six normal speakers and for three of the five stutterers. In the control groups, only one child suffered more speech interruptions by the end of the four-month experiment. Johnson believed his study proved that stuttering had its roots in social causes.

During World War II, some of Johnson's graduate students who knew about the study began calling it "the monster study." They suggested to Johnson that the public might compare it with Nazi experiments that were coming to light. Johnson therefore suppressed public acknowledgment of the study. Knowing the results he was able, however, to present other evidence to support his thesis. For example, he noted that some anthropologists found no stuttering, not even a word for the problem, in certain Native American tribes. His findings became widely accepted.

Meanwhile life worsened for several of the subjects. Two girls ran away from the orphanage but were caught and sent to state training school. Many years later, some subjects reported that stuttering ruined their lives, causing them to live as recluses. Others were able to overcome the stuttering for a while, only to have it recur later in their lives. To this day, Johnson's theory that positive reinforcement works best for children with speech difficulties is a dominant view. At age 84, Mary Tudor remains deeply conflicted about her role in the project. She has strong recollections of the "hard, terrible thing" she was doing to those children. Nevertheless, she says, "It was a small price to pay for science. Look at the countless number of children it helped."

Study Questions

1. How important does this research appear to be? What is its significance?

2. To what extent was deception a feature of this study, and is deception essential to obtaining information desired by the researcher?

3. How might this study have been designed to secure the desired information and not damage the children?

Adapted from Jim Dyer, "Ethics and Orphans: The 'Monster Study,'" *San Jose Mercury News,* June 10, 2001; and Jim Dyer, "Officials Apologize for Tests on Stuttering," *San Jose Mercury News,* June 13, 2001. See also Frank Silverman, "The 'Monster' Study," *Journal of Fluency Disorders* 1988 (13): 225–231.

3.14

Perinatal HIV Transmission Studies

United States policies require that all clinical trials sponsored by federal agencies abide by certain regulations. Critics maintain that those regulations sometimes hinder progress, and they demand more flexible standards. Large sections of the global community do not have reasonable hope of receiving the kind of medical care that is known to reduce the transmission of HIV infection between pregnant mothers and their children. As a result, researchers and countries gravely affected by AIDS tried to find cheap alternatives to expensive pharmaceutical products. This desperation led to studies that provoke controversy to this date. They raise important questions as to whether the studies amounted to an off-shore dumping of risk or whether people in other countries are entitled to make their own assessment of risks and benefits apart from rules of the United States government.

In the late 1990s researchers began a series of studies on ways to protect newborn children from their mother's AIDS-HIV infection. These studies were performed in Burkina Faso, the Ivory Coast, Thailand, and a number of other developing countries. They were supported through the U.S. Centers for Disease Control and Prevention (CDC), but to conduct them, sponsors had to apply for a waiver that would allow them to include a placebo arm. The goal was to find alternatives to the expensive course of AZT that is administered to pregnant women as a way of reducing the likelihood that their infants will be infected with HIV. This treatment is recommended by the CDC for all pregnant women in the United States with AIDS-HIV, and failure to adhere to it would open physicians in the United States to serious charges of malpractice.

Toward the end of finding less expensive treatments, researchers evaluated reduced dosages of AZT, injections of gamma globulin, vaginal washings, and other uncomplicated treatments. They believed that it was fair to perform these interventions against a placebo because treatment was virtually unavailable to women in these countries. In a sense, the existing standard of medical care for pregnant women with HIV was no treatment at all. In fact, researchers were granted the waiver from regulations that would require them to adhere to United States standards for clinical trials while doing research abroad. The trials also went forward with the approval of relevant public health agencies or ministries of host countries.

Critics insisted that these experimental interventions should be tested against the standard of care, namely, AZT. They regarded these studies as being of little benefit to the women involved, who were receiving either an intervention of unproved value or no treatment at all. Others saw exploitation in the motives of researchers who would shift the risks of experimentation offshore; no United States women were being asked to face the risks of unproved interventions.

The CDC responded by invoking guideline 8 of the International Guidelines for Biomedical Research Involving Human Subjects prepared by the Council for

International Organizations of Medical Sciences, which states, "Diseases that rarely or never occur in economically developed countries or communities exact a heavy toll of illness, disability, or death in some communities that are socially and economically at risk of being exploited for research purposes. Research into the prevention and treatment of such diseases is needed and, in general, must be carried out in large part in the countries and communities at risk."

Most critics were not persuaded, however, that anything of value was available to women in the trials. They feared that the subjects failed to understand what they were getting into because of poor informed consent processes and background problems of illiteracy and poverty. Others believed that even if the interventions did discover something of value, namely, the efficacy of a reduced course of AZT, that knowledge would benefit only people for whom AZT was already available. They contended that the only just clinical trials are those in which an experimental intervention is compared with standard therapy. Otherwise, the risk of exploitation is too great.

Study Questions

1. To what extent is the gravity of the AIDS epidemic sufficient justification for departing from standards the United States usually requires in its clinical trials?

2. Do you believe that the mechanisms for informed consent in the trials described could be adequate? Why or why not?

3. To what extent do you believe that the consent of countries involved in these trials is a defense against charges that these women were being exploited?

Adapted from David Weisstub, ed., *Research on Human Subjects: Ethics, Law and Social Policy* (Oxford: Pergamon, 1998), pp. 569–570. See also *Health Letter of the CDC* (1997, July 28): "CDC Explains Its Stand on Controversial Third World AZT Study," pp. 2–5; and Ronald Bayer, "Ethical Challenges of HIV Vaccine Trials in Less Developed Nations: Conflict and Consensus in the International Arena," *AIDS* 2000 (14) 8:1051–1057.

3.15

Payment for Research Subjects

In research involving healthy subjects, payment for subjects is the norm. For example, people can volunteer as subjects of sleep research in exchange for money. In research involving unhealthy people, such as cancer treatment studies, subjects are not paid for participating, although they may be provided a degree of medical care in addition to the intervention. Most commentary acknowledges that payment to subjects for therapeutic research may lead down a slippery slope, from inducement to coercion to unequal distribution of risks for poorer populations. Nevertheless, more and more subjects are being offered some compensation for being involved in research studies.

One standard for paying research subjects is the compensation model, according to which payment should be equal only to the costs of participation. Researchers may pay subjects at modest rates for travel costs, time, and so on, but not enough for subjects to make a profit. This model clearly avoids problems of undue influence over subjects.

Another standard is the market model, which holds that research subjects should be paid whatever is necessary to recruit them. When subjects are easy to recruit, they will be paid less than when subjects are harder to recruit. This model would probably be the most efficient, as it does not require that participants endure financial sacrifices to participate in research. On the contrary, subjects are motivated by the prospect of economic gain. However, commercialization of research may create professional volunteers who are vulnerable to exploitation. Compensating participants might also create unhealthy competition among researchers for subjects and raise the cost of research overall, thereby slowing progress.

The wage-payment model was proposed as an alternative to the other two. According to this model, all subjects would be paid standard rates on the theory that people performing similar functions should be treated similarly. What rate should this be? Participation in research ordinarily requires few skills, but it does require time, effort, and possibly uncomfortable procedures and undesirable side effects. Payment should therefore be on a par with unskilled but essential jobs. It would be a fairly low, hourly wage, but subjects could also receive bonuses if they participated in especially uncomfortable or burdensome interventions. This minimum wage would avoid problems of inducement, reduce competition for subjects among researchers, and promote equity in the treatment of subjects. Moreover, researchers would have an incentive to keep risks to subjects low in order to avoid paying bonuses.

Study Questions

1. What arguments can be put forward in favor of paying people for participating in clinical trials?

2. How convincing is the view that the market should decide how much subjects should be paid? That is, should people be offered as much as is necessary for them to agree to participate, or is there something about research that makes another standard of payment appropriate?

3. How convincing is the notion that participation in clinical trials is like low-skill work and therefore worthy only of a minimum wage?

Adapted from Neal Dickert, Christine Grady, "What's the Price of a Research Subject? Approaches to Payment for Research Participation," *New England Journal of Medicine* 1999 (341): 198–203.

3.16

Involvement of Poor and Wealthy Subjects

Research ethics developed mainly as a way to protect subjects from risk. Given this history, ethicists put a great deal of emphasis on informed consent, on the right to withdraw from studies, and on the use of vulnerable populations. A more recent trend in research ethics concerns equitable access by various groups to the benefits of research.

Adam Hislop, PharmD, was new to research. He had spent about ten years as a dispensing pharmacist, and was now teaching a course at a college of pharmacy where he also joined a senior pharmacist in a number of research projects. The senior investigator was on the verge of retirement and entrusted Hislop with the task of moving a small study of beta-blocking agents through the institution's IRB.

Hislop duly filled out the necessary forms and thought approval would be a mere formality. He was surprised to receive a letter stating that the proposal had not been approved because the IRB was concerned that subjects for the study were to be recruited from a clinic run by the city for the poor, whose patient population was almost all from racial minorities. The IRB was unsatisfied that the researchers offered no justification for choosing this patient population.

In fact, Hislop and his senior colleague had chosen the site because it was well known for its hypertension clinic, and they thought patients would be easy to recruit there. In resubmitting the proposal, Hislop decided that it would be easier to bypass the question of the use of vulnerable subjects. He made arrangements to conduct the study at another clinic in a pricey part of town. He expected the study might be completed faster there because of greater compliance with drug therapy. In addition, there would be no question of exploiting vulnerable patients.

Hislop was therefore surprised to receive a letter from the IRB questioning this new proposal. The board was worried that leaving out the poorer clinic meant that vulnerable populations might be excluded from potential benefits of the beta-blocker study. Dr. Hislop was thoroughly confused about what the IRB wanted.

Study Questions

1. Why would an IRB be concerned about the selection of a clinic catering primarily to racial minorities who are also poor?

2. How convincing is the IRB position that selection of a research site in a wealthy part of town denies possible benefits to the poor? Is it not true that studying this wealthy site would protect the poor from possible risks of the drugs under study?

3. What do you think the IRB was looking for in terms of access to the trial, protection from exploitation, and equitable distribution of risks and benefits? Would it be enough to conduct half the study at the city clinic and the rest at the wealthy clinic?

Adapted from Robert M. Veatch, Amy Haddad, *Case Studies in Pharmacy Ethics* (New York: Oxford University Press, 1999), p. 228.

Inclusion of Pregnant Women in Clinical Trials

The biomedical study of women raises concerns about the effect of experimental interventions on pregnant women and their fetuses. Pregnancy may alter the severity of some diseases, and fetuses and women may be put at risk through exposure to new drugs and devices. To protect against these risks, federal regulations limited the extent to which researchers could study new drugs and devices in pregnant women. This approach had the effect, however, of limiting knowledge about the best clinical care of women during pregnancy. Uneasiness over this effect led to new regulations in 2001, although it is not clear that all difficulties have been resolved.

In the 1960s and 1970s scandals involving unethical medical research led the Department of Health and Human Services in 1975 to put in place regulations governing vulnerable populations. Among these affected groups were pregnant women and fetuses, children, and women of reproductive age, all of whom were to be excluded from participation in phase I and early phase II clinical trials.

In January 2001, three days before the end of President Clinton's term, the DHHS issued an amendment to regulations governing participation of women in clinical research. The new rule purported to resolve legal and ethical ambiguities surrounding the inclusion of pregnant women. Specifically, it promised to alter the presumption of these pregnant women to one of including them and to "enhance . . . the opportunity for participation of pregnant women in research by promoting a policy of presumed inclusion. . . ." After brief suspension, these regulations took effect in 2002.

The regulation allows inclusion of pregnant women as long as "scientifically appropriate" preclinical studies were performed in pregnant animals and clinical studies in nonpregnant women, to provide data for assessing potential risks during pregnancy. In addition, the proposed study must pose no greater than minimal risk to the fetus. In the event of greater than minimal risk, a pregnant woman may be included only if the study is likely to "hold out the prospect of direct benefit for the woman or the fetus."

Study Questions

1. The goal of federal regulations is to protect research subjects. Do you believe that the original regulations took an appropriate approach to protecting fertile females, pregnant women, and fetuses from research risk? What was the effect of this approach?

2. The new regulation permits but does not require inclusion of pregnant women in clinical research. Do you believe that pharmaceutical manufacturers will be interested in increasing studies in pregnant women? What are the incentives? What are the obstacles?

3. Fear of legal liability leads researchers and sponsors to guard against participation of pregnant women in clinical research. Do you think that mechanisms to address this fear would

work to increase the role of women in clinical studies? Such mechanisms include, for example, caps on the liability sponsors would face, creation of a federal fund to compensate harmed subjects, and building liability costs into the costs of doing business. Should one or more of these mechanisms be put in place to increase involvement of pregnant women in clinical trials?

Adapted from unpublished work by Michelle Oberman, JD, MPH, Timothy F. Murphy, PhD, Joel Frader, MD.

4

Conflicts of Interest

Introduction

A conflict of interest is a situation in which someone has a private or personal interest that could influence or appear to influence the way in which that person makes decisions and carries out professional duties. In other words, people could make decisions to benefit themselves and not the institutions or individuals they are obliged to serve. Conflicts of interest often involve financial interests, but they may also extend to other domains such as professional prestige, social status, and public visibility. In research, conflicts of interest can work against the integrity of science and can undermine the protection of research subjects. They occur when researchers' interests diverge from the requirements of objectivity, professional conduct, and the obligation to protect the safety and well-being of subjects. For both practical and moral reasons, it is important to identify and control conflicts of interests in research.

Disadvantages to Science from Conflicts of Interest
In scientific research, conflicts of interest can put the integrity of data and interpretations at risk. Researchers may be tempted to deviate from objective standards in

reporting and interpreting data in order to produce outcomes that are favorable to sponsors or that may advance their own interests.

Sponsorship   The source of funds can raise certain conflicts of interest with respect to objectivity. For example, a tobacco company can pay the salary of researchers studying the long-term health risks of cigarettes, cigars, and snuff. Or, the manufacturer of a breast implant can pay for a study of its health risks. If the results seem to be unfavorable as the studies progress, the sponsors may withdraw financial support. If the studies show that these products do damage health, the sponsors may decline to publish the research. To cite another example, researchers may not wish to antagonize their financial sponsors, and thus may be tempted to report data from studies in ways that minimize health risks associated with products. Companies are free, of course, to sponsor their own research, but to control undue influence most scientific journals have in place mechanisms that require the disclosure of financial sponsorship and affiliations. At the very least, this disclosure lets readers evaluate study conclusions in relation to possible goals of the sponsor. In this way, the objectivity of data is not assumed without question.

In one rather telling turn of events, a prestigious medical journal had to change a conflict of interest policy. The *New England Journal of Medicine* once refused to publish review articles of drugs by writers with financial ties to pharmaceutical companies that manufactured those drugs. The journal could not find enough qualified independent authors, however, and therefore relaxed its standard. It will now publish these papers as long as the authors do not receive more than $10,000 a year from a drug company in speaking and consulting fees.[1] The policy does not reject articles if the author receives this total amount from more than one company. In effect, the journal tried to find reviewers without financial ties on the theory that these reviewers could be more objective than others. Corporate sponsorship of research is far-reaching, however, and the journal concluded that limited financial ties to industry do not stand in the way of objective evaluation.

Lawyers who sued the University of Pennsylvania after the 1999 death of eighteen-year-old Jesse Gelsinger drew a great deal of attention to the way in which the trial that enrolled the young man was funded. The study was sponsored by and carried out at the Institute for Human Gene Therapy at the university.[2] Among other charges, the lawsuit noted that Dr. James Wilson founded Genovo, which in turned funded the Institute for Human Gene Therapy of which he was director. Funding apparently took the form of stock transfers and agreements on patents and licensing. The institute funded the bioethics center from which Dr. Wilson sought counsel about enrolling subjects. In short, there was a tangle of financial interests, and the lawsuit alleged that Jesse Gelsinger was improperly enrolled, in part, because of judgments exercised to protect those financial interests. The litigants reached an agreement out of court so that these allegations were never fully explored at trial.

It is an open question, however, whether such financial arrangements can influence judgments in a way that are prejudicial to subjects.

Disadvantages to Subjects from Conflicts of Interest

An imbalance often exists between researchers and subjects when it comes to understanding a study. Biomedical research often involves exposure to risks, and conflicts of interest on the part of researchers, who are in a position to gain financially if a drug under study succeeds, for example, may lead them to minimize those risks when explaining research to potential subjects. Comparatively naive subjects are in no position to judge that it will be the researcher who has more to gain than themselves. Yet an enthusiastic recommendation from the researcher may induce them to participate whereas a more circumspect description would cause them to hesitate or decline. Because subjects are vulnerable, researchers' ulterior motives can be suspect as they try to enroll subjects quickly and easily, whether or not involvement may be in the subjects' best interests. At worst, researchers might attempt to exploit subjects for their own gain; at minimum it can appear that researchers are guilty of wrongful inducement to enroll subjects.

Physician-researchers often receive considerable sums of money for enrolling subjects in trials of new drugs. This is known as a capitation fee. If a physician receives, for example, $3,000 for enrolling a single subject, a real economic incentive exists to enroll as many subjects as possible. This money is sometimes restricted in its use. Depending on institutional policies, it cannot always be considered disposable income, but it may be used for office supplies, traveling to professional meetings, and so on. Whatever the rules are, incentives are strong to bring in as much money as possible in this way. It is an open question whether and to what extent capitation fees create conflicts of interest, especially when they are not disclosed to subjects.

The incentive of capitation fees should be contrasted with the way in which some people use experimental trials as their source of medical care: those who are not able to pay for medical care look to research trials as a source of treatment. These circumstances—researchers looking for hefty capitation fees, subjects looking for free medical care—may represent the worst possible collision of interests. The existence of well-formulated inclusion and exclusion criteria—who is eligible to participate and who is not—can help protect against the most harmful effects of this collision.

Clinical Care

At times the very goals of a trial may seem to be in conflict with a subject's best interest. For example, it is in every person's best interest to avoid HIV infection. No reasonable person could prefer to be infected with HIV, yet vaccine research depends on people being exposed to the virus, otherwise the effect of experimental vaccines will remain unknown. Because the consequences of the infection are so devastating, it would be immoral to ask vaccine subjects to behave *as if they were immune* and expose themselves to HIV. But, again, if people do not expose

themselves, no one will know whether or not the vaccine works. Does this ambiva-
lence—wanting to protect from HIV but needing exposure to it—put researchers in
a conflict of interest?

In this instance, to avoid conflict of interest researchers have an ethical obligation
both to administer the experimental vaccine and to educate people against behavior
that might expose them to HIV infection. Despite education and their best intentions,
some people will fail to avoid sexual behaviors and needle use that expose them to
HIV. Moreover, people may wrongly believe that the vaccine is fully effective and
continue to act irresponsibly. The vaccine will be tested, therefore, *despite* counsel and
education by researchers. On its face, it might be seen as a conflict of interest to ask
subjects to enroll in an anti-HIV vaccine trial, but interest in testing the vaccine is offset
by counsel and education about ways to protect against HIV exposure. After all, by
entering the trial subjects will receive education about preventing HIV that they might
not have received otherwise. They may therefore even be at an advantage over others
in protecting themselves from infection, whether or not they benefit from the vaccine.

It would be worrisome in the extreme, however, if education about HIV risks
were colored by a conflict of interest. For example, potential subjects who believed
that the vaccine would in fact protect them ("Why else would the doctors give it to
me?") should probably be excluded from participation. It would be a manifest conflict of interest for researchers to enroll people who misunderstood the unproved
state of the vaccine and who would therefore take no action to protect themselves
against exposure to HIV. This example shows that ways are available to resolve
tensions between what researchers want to learn (whether a vaccine works) and what
subjects want to have (protection against infection).

Controlling Conflicts of Interest

In one sense potential conflicts of interest are so much a part of the research landscape as to seem inescapable. Background considerations are always present that
can color the researcher's interest in enrolling this subject right now rather than
someone else later. These general considerations involve the successful performance
of one's job, promotions, tenure in academic settings, prestige, honors and awards,
future grants, and so on. Indeed, even if researchers have no special financial incentive to succeed—they will still receive their annual salary from their university—
they may still derive enormous pride and social prestige from doing advanced work
at the very frontiers of medicine. In short, researchers may stand to gain in a way
that goes against a dispassionate and objective assessment of whether a particular
study is in the best interest of a particular subject. Nevertheless, some conflicts of
interest are more egregious than others, and methods should be—and are—in place
to control their worst possible effects.

To control possible bias in publication, journals often require researchers to disclose funding sources of their work as a way of keeping conflicts of interest in check.
These journals then determine whether or not these sources should be identified in

the publication. At some journals, this disclosure is a matter of editorial judgment. Others require disclosure with publication as a matter of course. Some universities and colleges have taken steps to limit the degree of financial involvement a researcher can have with the sponsor of a drug or device under study. They forbid, for example, owning stock above a particular monetary level.

At the present time, discussion suggests that to control conflicts of interest greater disclosure to subjects of researchers' financial relationship to research is necessary. As part of the informed consent process, should researchers disclose, for example, that they or their institutions will receive a capitation fee for enrolling subjects? Should researchers be required to disclose that they own stock in a company that produces the drug or device under study? Should they be required to disclose that they are officers of the corporation that is developing the drug or device? Answers to these questions are not well formulated at present, and they deserve much more analysis.

One ethicist recommended that universities stop using profits from research altogether and establish themselves as truly nonprofit institutions.[3] He suggested that indirect costs generate potential conflicts of interest. Universities charge sponsors of research, the federal government included, for support of the university-research environment. In theory this money goes to cover electricity, heating, building maintenance, and other overhead costs. Given that funds for indirect costs are an important source of revenue for institutions, it is unclear if anything will ever come of this recommendation.

When it comes to IRB review of research, federal regulations work against conflicts of interest. Board members who conduct research may not sit in judgment of their own work. They may be present for discussion of the work if the IRB wishes their input, but they are not entitled to vote in favor (or against for that matter) their own study. Other members of the IRB act as impartial judges, not the researchers who have a strong interest in projects being approved.[4]

To be sure, research will always struggle with potential conflicts of interest because it has many functions in this society and because lines between universities and industry continue to blur. Nevertheless, disclosure of financial interests, and possibly other interests of the researcher, can help subjects decide whether to enroll in research and clarify the interpretation researchers put on their findings. Sometimes disclosure will not be enough, and certain researchers should abstain from projects that are manifestly open to distortions rooted in their own financial and professional gain.

References

1. John McKenzie, "Conflict of Interest? Medical Journal Changes Policy of Finding Independent Doctors to Write," ABCNews.com, June 12, 2002.

2. http://www.sskrplaw.com/links/healthcare2.html.

3. Baruch Brody, *The Ethics of Biomedical Research: An International Perspective* (New York: Oxford University Press, 1998).

4. 45 C.F.R. 46 Sec. 107.

The John Moore Case

This landmark case deals with the interests and rights donors have with regard to tissues and other bodily substances used for research and commercial purposes. The case moved through a variety of courts, and although it established a standard about informed consent and donor rights, it is unclear that it will be the last word on donor interests because it remains controversial. Nevertheless, in many ways it sets the terms of the debate as it is argued today.

In 1976 Dr. David W. Golde began treating John Moore for hairy cell leukemia at the University of California at Los Angeles (UCLA). In the course of treatment Moore's spleen was removed. Moore had signed a consent form for the surgery, which noted that removed materials would be disposed of by cremation. In fact, pathological analysis of the tissue showed that it had interesting scientific properties, and Dr. Golde used the tissue without Moore's knowledge or consent to produce a cell line that reproduces itself indefinitely.

The cell line was used to produce nine pharmaceutically significant substances, including granulocyte–macrophage colony-stimulating factor. In 1984 this factor was patented by UCLA, and Golde established contracts for use of the cell line with a Boston company, giving him stock interests worth perhaps as much as $3 million. The Swiss pharmaceutical company Sandoz reportedly paid $15 million for the right to develop the cell line.

From 1976 to 1983, physicians continued to take substances from Moore: bone marrow, sperm, skin, and blood. They represented their actions as important for monitoring the man's medical condition, and provided no compensation. Moore became suspicious that he was being used for purposes other than medical treatment.

In April 1983, Moore was given a consent form that authorized research on his bodily tissues. He signed the document, but it made no mention of the use of his samples for commercial purposes. In September 1983, UCLA offered Moore a third consent form, asking him to waive any and all rights to cell line and products that might be developed from his cell line. Moore agreed to the removal of blood for research purposes, but expressly denied UCLA commercial rights to his cells.

Commercial use of his cell line continued, however, and in September 1984 Moore filed suit claiming malpractice and damages related to unauthorized use of property. The case went through various courts until reaching the California Supreme Court. That court held that Moore was wronged insofar his physician did not advise him about the nature or disposition of materials taken from his body. It did not, however, uphold his claim that his property interests had been damaged. He received no monetary settlement.

The court specifically went out of its way to say that acknowledging a property interest would slow research by wiping out economic incentives for researchers. The court also pointed out that acknowledging a property interest could mire researchers in lawsuits. Some agreed, saying that federal law was required to prohibit patients and research subjects from selling their tissues and cells, or making money from products derived from these substances. They maintained that a free market in tissue-cell research works against the development of an energetic biotech industry.

Study Questions

1. To what extent, if any, does it appear that John Moore was deceived about the use of biological materials taken from him?

2. Do you believe that Mr. Moore is entitled to decide whether or not biological materials taken from him in the course of medical care should be used for research? Why should these materials not be treated as biological waste?

3. In making its decision, the California Supreme Court held that to give Moore a property interest would slow scientific research and commercial development. In fact, the court did recognize biological materials as property; it simply held that they were not Moore's property. Do you agree with the logic of this decision?

Adapted from Ernest D. Prentice, John C. Wiltse, John G. Sharp, Dean L. Antonson, "An Institutional Policy on the Right to Benefit from the Commercialization of Human Biological Material," *Law, Medicine & Health Care* 1990 (18): 162–167; and Dorothy Nelkin, Lori B. Andrews, "Homo Economicus: Commercialization of Body Tissue in the Age of Biotechnology," *Hastings Center Report* 1998 (28): 30–39.

Compensation for Biological Materials

A precedent in law requires that donors be advised as to what may happen to tissues they donate. It does not require, however, that people who agree to give their tissues for study and development be compensated. Some donors may be compensated in minor ways, but no policy or custom returns benefit to people whose tissues are used to develop commercial products. In the following case, a major medical center discussed its reasons for declining to offer monetary compensation.

Genomic technology has substantially increased the demand for human tissue, both diseased and normal specimens. Dr. Barry Eisenstein, vice president for science and technology at Beth Israel Deaconess Medical Center in Boston, has said, "The value of patients' tissues has potentially gone up enormously." Nevertheless, that medical center turned away a family who was demanding a huge sum of money for samples of their tissues. The family members lived to great ages, and a gerontologist wanted to study them for a gene that might be responsible for their longevity.

The medical center defended its decision in a number of ways. Officials were uncomfortable paying this family while other families were donating tissues free of charge. They respected the view that tissue donation ought to be a matter of altruism, even as they admitted that it might be reasonable to offer compensation in some cases. In the main, though, they worried that compensation might produce inappropriate incentives. They also noted that paying for blood was more likely to result in hepatitis-infected blood than donations made without compensation. Finally, paying people for tissue could interfere with downstream commercial development. They noted that the court determined that John Moore did not have a monetary stake in his donated tissues and that this decision relied heavily on fear of obstacles for further commercial development.

That said, one official acknowledged that the medical center might have come to a different conclusion about compensation had there been an advocacy group that could have made more effective demands than a single family was able to do.

Commenting on the general expectation that donors receive no payment for their donations, Robert Cook-Deegan, a professor at the Georgetown University Kennedy Institute of Ethics, said, "We have a system where the research participants are treated as pure altruists, but everyone else is treated as a pure capitalist. I don't think that's quite fair."

Study Questions

1. How convincing is it that donors of biological materials should be compensated in only modest ways, for example, reimbursement for time and travel or small gifts?

2. Given that development of commercial products depends on the ingenuity and skill of researchers, isn't it fair to say that researchers ought to reap the rewards of their ingenuity, not donors, who could have done nothing with their biological materials in any case?

3. Is it possible to imagine a system of payment that would return some economic benefit to donors but not also kill the incentive of researchers to produce commercially valuable products? How, if at all, might such a system operate?

Adapted from Ted T. Ashburn, Sharon K. Wilson, Barry I. Eistenstein, "Human Tissue Research in the Genomic Era of Medicine," *Archives of Internal Medicine* 2000 (160): 3377–3384; and Gina Kolata, "Sharing of Profits Is Debated as the Value of Tissue Rises," *New York Times*, May 15, 2000.

Payments to Physicians for Enrolling Research Subjects

When physicians enroll patients in drug studies they can receive a per-subject fee of $2,000 to $5,000. This money, which functions as a kind of finder's fee, is usually put toward professional costs. Whereas subjects do not usually receive a comparable fee, they may receive free medical care associated with the study. Some worry about the propriety of these fees because of their potential to subordinate the subject's interests to the physician's financial gain.

Randall Erst is a physician in private practice and receives $3,000 for every patient he enrolls in a cancer drug study. If he enrolls a sufficient number of patients he will garner a substantial profit for his medical practice. Some of this money he will use to hire help to carry out the study.

Dr. Erst explains the availability of the research trial to a long-time patient and prospective subject, Mandy Vance. He tells Mr. Vance how this treatment would be different from treatment he would ordinarily receive. He explains that the new drug is promising, and that it and related medical care will be free. Dr. Erst mentions, too, the possibility that Mr. Vance might be assigned to the control group and thus would receive standard drug treatment rather than the experimental agent. Trusting the medical judgment of Dr. Erst, Mr. Vance decides to enroll in the study. He is glad that his medical care will be completely free, because he lacks health insurance. Dr. Erst does not mention the $3000 he will receive if Mr. Vance agrees to enroll in the study.

Study Questions

1. What harms might come about because of capitation payments made to physicians for enrolling subjects in research trials?

2. Those who defend the present system of physician payment for research contend that physician professionalism is an effective safeguard of the patient's interest. Do you believe that physician-researchers are trustworthy as a class, that they can be trusted not to jeopardize the well-being of their patients?

3. Critics of the status quo state that disclosure of payments to physicians gives patients one key piece of information necessary to help them judge whether physicians are acting in their own interests. Do you believe this line of reasoning to be convincing?

For more information see David S. Shimm, Roy G. Spece, Jr., Michelle Burpeau DiGregorio, "Conflicts of Interest in Relationships between Physicians and the Pharmaceutical Industry," in Roy G. Spece, Jr., David S. Shimm, Allen E. Buchanan, eds., *Conflicts of Interest in Clinical Practice and Research* (New York: Oxford University Press, 1996), pp. 321–357.

4.4

Conflict of Interest: Divesting Financial Interest

Professional societies are devoted to the interests of a particular scientific field and its members. As such, they do not have the power to establish laws or regulatory policy. Nevertheless, virtually all of them offer ethical advisories about how members should conduct themselves. Some urge researchers to avoid relationships with commercial sponsors, if such relationships would cloud their professional judgment.

In 2000 the American Society of Gene Therapy (ASGT) noted that federal guidelines attempt to reduce conflicts of interest by limiting the financial stake researchers can have in sponsoring companies. These guidelines limit involvement of researchers who have "significant financial interest" in such companies. They define significant financial interest as equity ownership of 5 percent or more, or payments that exceed more than $10,000 per year from that company.

The ASGT believed it was important to protect the best interest of patients in clinical trials. To that end, "clinical investigators must be able to design and carry out clinical research studies in an objective and unbiased manner, free from conflicts caused by significant financial involvement with the commercial sponsors of the study." They called on their members to abide by all relevant federal and institutional regulations for avoiding conflicts of interest.

In addition, the ASGT urged that all members of a research team—those involved in selection, informed consent, and medical management of subjects—be free of equity, stock options, or comparable financial arrangements in clinical trials. This recommendation exceeds existing federal requirements. In any case, the society urged its members who currently had such arrangements to discontinue them.

Study Questions

1. Many researchers have financial interests in corporations that sponsor biomedical research. What are ways in which these interests may influence their decisions when conducting studies?

2. Financial interests that researchers have generally are trivial in the sense that they are extremely unlikely to sway professional judgments. Do you believe that recommendations with regard to ownership and payment are sufficient to protect professional judgment? Are the numbers too high, too low, or just right?

3. The only mechanism of enforcement available to the ASGT if one of its members violates this advisory is to drop the researcher from membership, which is voluntary to begin with. What other mechanisms might be available to protect against financial conflicts of interest?

From American Society of Gene Therapy (www.asgt.org/policy/).

Research on the Maltreatment of Children

In all states, health professionals, teachers, and police are required to report sus-
pected child abuse and neglect to legal and social service authorities. Researchers
sometimes face situations that open them to civil or criminal liability if they do not
disclose such activities that cares to light during studies. However, these disclosures
can interfere with research because subjects may not trust the researchers, and dis-
trust could alter their behavior. Subjects might even avoid the researchers altogether.
Dilemmas therefore arise between securing the trust of participants and making dis-
closures that have serious effects for them.

LONGSCAN is a federally sponsored study of the determinants and effects of child
maltreatment. It involves the long-term study of children ranging in age from
newborns to early adulthood. Among other things, the study hopes to examine
the impact of maltreatment on children's development, school performance, peer
relationships, aggressiveness, dating and mating behaviors, and attitudes about
parenting.

Participants were recruited from families reported to the authorities in various
jurisdictions for suspected abuse, maltreatment, or neglect, depending on laws in
force in those locations. Some were recruited because their children had received
particular medical diagnoses (e.g., failure to thrive). Control subjects were also entered into the study.

Both parents and children were studied. For children up to age six, the mother
was the primary respondent. Researchers interviewed children age six and over for
certain data. After a child reached the age of twelve, researchers took data primarily
from them. In fact, these children were asked to assent to participate. Researchers
also examined social service records to determine whether agencies had intervened
in response to allegations of maltreatment.

To avoid the duty to report possible criminal behavior or behavior that would
trigger involvement of social service agencies, researchers asked about indirect indicators of maltreatment. They asked parents, for example, about disciplining their children. They also asked parents and children about stresses, family circumstances, and
so on. The informed consent process advised participants that the researchers had
duties to report maltreatment as defined by law. It also advised that if participants
disclosed clear maltreatment, they would in fact make that report. However, when
researchers asked mothers if their children age eight or over had ever been sexually
abused, they did not seek the identity of alleged abusers if the mothers said yes.

At age twelve, the children were asked about neglect and abuse using a computer
program. Some answers were encrypted in a way that stripped all identifying information from respondents. Nevertheless, if children did make incriminating statements, researchers would report severe, life-threatening abuse. However, they

decided not to report old or trivial abuse, reports that in their opinion were unlikely to lead to action by social service agencies. They termed these "nuisance reports." The researchers hold a federal certificate of confidentiality that protects them from legal liability for failing to disclose information they obtain in the course of a study. These certificates are issued to researchers who must gain the trust of participants who may worry about exposure to legal action.

Study Questions

1. What is the key conflict in this area of research, and why is it an ethical dilemma?

2. Do you think that need to foster trust with participants justifies researchers' decision not to disclose certain allegations of child maltreatment?

3. Do you believe that children at age twelve can be advised in a meaningful way that if they make allegations of maltreatment (including by parents) that reports must be filed and that families may be broken apart as a result?

4. Some believe that *all* allegations of maltreatment should be reported, and therefore, research of the kind involved in LONGSCAN should not be permitted. What is the reason for such a view, and how convincing is it?

Adapted from Desmond K. Runyan, "Maltreatment in Families: A Research Dilemma," in Nancy M.P. King, Gail A. Henderson, Jane Stein, eds. *Beyond Regulations: Ethics in Human Subjects Research* (Chapel Hill: University of North Carolina Press, 1999) pp. 161–170. See also http://www.sph.unc.edu/iprc/longscan/.

Artificial Hearts: How Many Tries?

The question of when an intervention is ready to go forward is always problematic, and this was especially true in the case of artificial hearts. The field of human heart transplantation was not well developed as researchers tried to find mechanical devices that could serve as permanent or temporary implantable blood pumps. In the following case, the question of how many times a device should be tried is raised pointedly by the way transplantation affects quality of life. However, new innovations often fail many times before they succeed, raising important ethical questions about consent and protection of patients.

Barney Clark was born in 1921 and, after a lifetime of smoking, was diagnosed in 1978 with emphysema, congestive heart failure, and cardiomyopathy (degeneration of heart tissue). Heart transplantation was relatively new at that time, and Clark at 57 was considered too old to be eligible for the surgery.

A medical committee at the University of Utah was interested in finding a candidate to be the first person to receive an artificial heart, the Jarvik-7 (named after its designer). This committee thought that the candidate should be so ill that death was imminent and the prognosis offered no more than a year of life. Clark met these conditions.

Clark signed an eleven-page consent form, he was interviewed by members of the IRB about his choice, and a team of physicians tried to test his determination by urging him to change his mind. He did not.

Dr. William DeVries led the medical team that supervised implantation of the artificial heart in a complicated surgery that began at 11 p.m. December 1, 1982. The Jarvik-7 was a mechanical device that was hooked by tubes to an external air compressor to move blood. The external compressor weighed 375 pounds, and Clark could never be without it. After the operation, Clark was in a poor state and experienced considerable confusion, delirium, memory loss, periods of semiconsciousness, and seizures. He required surgical intervention to replace one of the heart valves which broke two weeks after the initial operation.

Clark's health was never especially good, but he did appear before videocameras, and selectively edited interviews were released to the media. This public visibility gave the impression that he was glad to be alive. In fact, Clark's overall condition could only be called burdensome, and he died on March 23, 1983, of multiple organ failure. It was not long before scientists were split in their opinion about the value of the artificial heart. Some called it one of the boldest experiments ever attempted. Others said it more than failed. Still others called it unacceptably expensive. DeVries defended the artificial heart noting that, without it, Clark would have been dead by midnight on December 1, 1982.

The FDA, which oversees medical devices, allowed DeVries three more tries with the Jarvik-7. The first of these patients died after surviving for twenty-one months;

the second survived for ten months and two days; the third survived ten days. In the last case, DeVries admitted that the surgery had probably shortened the patient's life. In 1990 the FDA withdrew approval for use of the Jarvik-7 as a permanent device, or even as a bridge for a patient awaiting a human heart transplant. Patient referrals to DeVries dropped, because other physicians were concerned that he had too many conflicts of interest rooted in his desire for success and financial gain. They worried that he was putting technical success ahead of patient care.

Study Questions

1. To what extent is it ethical for a health care team to offer a patient an intervention that might possibly extend his life and then try and persuade him not to accept it?

2. What information do you think would be crucial in explaining the risks and benefits of an artificial heart implant?

3. It is reasonable to expect some failure with new medical interventions. In your view, do the survival times of the patients in this case amount to a reason to shut down the use of a mechanical heart, or should more attempts be allowed?

Adapted from Gregory E. Pence, *Classic Cases in Medical Ethics* (New York: McGraw-Hill 1990), pp. 299–309.

Conflict of Interest: Institutional Financial Gain

Most discussions of conflict of interest focus on the financial involvement of individual investigators. The question arises whether a physician is motivated in treating a patient in the best way possible or in a way that advances his or her own interests. One bioethicist challenges the research community to consider the way in which institutional benefit might also be implicated in conflict of interest.

One of the main reasons for worrying about conflict of interest is that it may contribute to fraud and misconduct in research. However, there is another worry: conflict of interest may lead to poor judgment when designing and implementing research studies.

Various measures are in place to try and curb the worst conflicts of interest; however, most are focused on explicit financial arrangements between sponsors of research and people who actually carry out the studies. This focus assumes that commercial conflicts of interest are the only ones worth worrying about.

Conflicts of interest can occur outside commercial arrangements in both public and private universities. These institutions often have a great deal at stake when administrators and IRBs make judgments about research carried out there. For example, institutions have considerable influence when choosing the kinds of research to be pursued, sources of funding, and subjects to be enrolled. Grants are a major source of income for universities, and pressure to maintain strong research programs is substantial.

"Profits to individuals or institutions from grants can be just as much a source of conflict of interest as equity holdings or consultancy fees, and we need to control the former as much as the latter."

One way to control undue influence of this pressure is to make sure that grants cover only the cost of doing research. It may be difficult to know exactly how much it costs to run a study, but universities should strive to achieve a nonprofit standard when seeking funding. If they do not, they risk running afoul of poor judgment in the design and conduct of trials involving human subjects.

Study Questions

1. Conflicts of interest arise when researchers are in the position of making decisions that benefit them, as against their institutions or subjects. Is disclosure of financial interests always enough to protect against the worst effects of conflicts of interest?

2. Universities in the United States are heavily dependent on grant money for their operations. Baruch Brody believes that an institution's use of research money from a federal agency has the same potential for conflict of interest as use of money from corporations. Is it convincing to say that universities are in positions of conflict of interest because of their reliance on grant funds from federal and nonprofit sources? How might one know if this is true or not?

3. Would it be appropriate for universities to run as true nonprofits and accept only as much money as is absolutely necessary to run particular studies?

Adapted from Baruch Brody, *Ethical Issues in Drug Testing, Approval, and Pricing: The Clot-Dissolving Drugs* (New York: Oxford University Press, 1995), pp. 144–152.

4.8

Independence and Sponsorship of IRBs

The Code of Federal Regulations specifies the composition and responsibilities of IRBs. The study of how those boards function is not well developed. Oversight agencies tend to look at their compliance with certain regulations rather than to evaluate the way in which they function individually and as a whole.

To function effectively, an IRB has to have a good working relationship with its institution. It must understand the environment and the subjects it is likely to enroll in studies. Because of this close working relationship, the IRB can come to see itself as an agent of the institution rather than as, say, a body representing either the community or federal government.

An IRB may look favorably on research proposals that come from certain departments or that are sponsored by particular individuals. Some boards may not wish to slow a university's goal of achieving substantial increases in grant support. As a result, they, or some of their members, may be tempted to facilitate approval of certain projects. Boards may also be predisposed to recruiting particular subjects known to them through personal ties.

If IRBs can be influenced to favoritism in their reviews of research proposals, their judgment can go the other way too. They may have an unfavorable opinion of certain departments or researchers and be inclined to resist proposals coming from those sources.

In short, because IRBs have an intimate connection with sponsoring universities or institutions, their judgment as independent evaluators of studies can come into question. Whether indirect factors such as prestige, institutional income, and institutional loyalty influence board decisions is not well studied.

Study Questions

1. In practice, many members of a university IRB do come from the university itself. In fact, federal regulations require members who are familiar with the institution where research will be carried out. How desirable is it to have IRBs independent from sponsoring institutions?

2. At the present time, federal regulations require that one member of the IRB come from the community and not the sponsoring institution. Do you believe that community representation is adequate to ensure that these boards do not make poor judgments in reviewing research proposals?

3. What might an IRB do to achieve more independence from its sponsoring institution?

Capitation Fees for Research Subjects

Some studies involve capitation costs paid to the researchers. In large studies, this money can quickly add up to considerable amounts. As the hypothetical case below indicates, ethical questions arise about whether this money raises conflicts of interest for the researcher.

Felix Cannon, PharmD, was explaining capitation to his new associate, Heloise Gato, PharmD. Gato was joining Cannon in a study of an antiemetic drug, and he was encouraging her to identify patients at the local medical center who would be good subjects. He and Gato will receive $3,000 in capitation for each subject they enroll, to a maximum of fifty patients over the next year. After expenses, those fees could create a surplus of $118,000.

When Gato asked how the money would be spent, Cannon explained that it would be used to hire someone to manage the data and to cover medical costs associated with the study. It also could be applied to travel to professional meetings, equipment, supplies, and to help run other unfunded studies. The medical center might take part of the money as a "tax" for overhead, but the rest could be used for professional purposes. Cannon explained that at the beginning of the study each patient would receive $100 for filling out a ten-page questionnaire about diet and symptoms.

Study Questions

1. What are the points at which a desire to generate capitation fees might impair physician judgment? What kind of evaluation would show that some aspect of physician judgment was influenced by money from a trial's sponsor?

2. Are you convinced that capitation payments researchers receive should be disclosed as part of the informed consent process? What would a subject gain from this disclosure?

Adapted from Robert M. Veatch, Amy Haddad, *Case Studies in Pharmacy Ethics* (New York: Oxford University Press, 1999), pp. 230–231.

4.10

Research Universities for Hire?

Universities increasingly pursue funding from commercial sources, as well as commercial relationships with the private sector. They also act as commercial operations in their own right. In the past, concerns were raised that corporate sponsorship of research can raise conflicts of interest with regard to what is researched, what results are published, when results are published (if at all), and who is employed. These worries intensified when the Bayh-Dole Act of 1980 permitted universities to profit from research funded at taxpayer expense. Many universities now have offices of technology development whose purpose is to generate such profits.

In 1999 Novartis, a Swiss pharmaceutical corporation, announced an agreement with the University of California at Berkeley to support basic research in its Department of Plant and Microbial Biology. In exchange for $25 million, the university would turn the licensing rights to approximately one-third of its discoveries over to the company. This arrangement would also extend to discoveries made with the support of government dollars. Using public funds to generate private benefit is in fact permitted by the Bayh–Dole Act, intended to give universities an incentive to create more useful inventions. The act is based on the concept that universities would be better than the government at bringing products to market. Another aspect of the agreement was that two Novartis representatives would become members of the department research committee that decides how the department's money is spent.

Various protests met the Novartis-Berkeley deal. The chief criticism was that the collaboration amounted to a betrayal of the role of the university as a center of free intellectual inquiry. Critics saw threats to basic research as against research having an immediate commercial application. They also saw the university as becoming a collaborator in the capitalist process, rather than an impartial judge. Some professors complained that the arrangement undercut their rights of free speech. Others worried that the ultimate benefactors of research would be funders rather than the public. The arrangement might slow the sharing of basic scientific ideas, samples, and results.

The dean of the College of Natural Sciences at Berkeley defended the arrangement, in part by saying that the money could be used elsewhere on the campus, especially to modernize outdated buildings. He also observed that government support for university research had been diminishing. Without this money, he saw no other way to keep Berkeley in the vanguard of research.

Study Questions

1. What conflicts of interest might the arrangement between Novartis and the University of California either cause or appear to cause?

2. One of the benefits of a separation between universities and researchers is that university researchers are often in the position to offer disinterested evaluation of medical drugs and devices. Do you believe that the arrangement described here dilutes the university's capacity to offer such independent evaluations?

3. Given the involvement of two representatives, Novartis has a say in how department funds are spent. Concerns were raised about turning the department into an extension of the corporation. Could these concerns be kept in check if the Novartis representatives could participate only as consultants and not as actual decision makers?

Adapted from Eyal Press, Jennifer Washburn, "The Kept University," *Atlantic Monthly*, March 2000, pp. 39–54.

4.11

The Function of IRBs

Federal regulations make clear that IRBs should focus on the ethical protections of the research projects they examine, not their long-term social implications. For example, IRBs should not concern themselves with the likely social impact of a drug if the drug would be costly to patients in the future. At times, however, researchers raise questions about the value of particular projects, wondering if it is ethical to ask subjects to be involved in trials of agents without proved significance.

Freida Belton is a clinical psychologist who sits on a university IRB. The board has received a request to review a proposed study examining the way men and women in their seventies talk about unpleasant things that occurred in their lives.

The subjects will be told that the name of the project is "A Study of Recollections," but they will not specifically be told that it will be about painful memories. In fact, the researchers plan to ask men and women to identify the worst things that ever happened to them: the death of a child or parent, domestic violence, wartime experience, and so on. The study will then analyze the narrative format of the answers. For example, do they use the passive voice ("I was hit by my father") or the active voice ("My father hit me")? Do they speak in the first person ("I was a happy child before that time") or collectively ("We were all happy children in those days")? The researchers hypothesize that the way seniors structure their experiences verbally can help them cope with these experiences emotionally.

Professor Belton knows about this area of research and believes it to be a colossal waste of time. She thinks that most work done in this field has no clinical value and will never lead to any. She thinks many more important questions deserve to be answered about the emotional well-being of seniors, rather than wondering how they phrase their painful memories. She is tempted to encourage other IRB members to vote against the proposal. Even if she cannot persuade them that the study is not worthwhile, she thinks they will accept her view that it is deceptive.

Study Questions

1. To what extent does this study involve deception? Is the title justified in terms of the actual goals and methods?

2. Is Professor Belton justified in her belief that the IRB should not accept the study because she thinks it will have no value? Is she justified in opposing the study, or are her views about the research so strong that she should excuse herself from discussing or voting on the proposal?

3. What changes might make the protocol more acceptable to Professor Belton? Is it possible to reduce risks to the subjects?

For-Profit IRBs

Most IRBs that conduct ethics reviews of government-sponsored research are composed of volunteers. Members generally receive no compensation for participating. In some cases, they may receive very small benefits, such as meals when meetings occur at particular times of the day, or small stipends. Federal regulations do not exclude the possibility of for-profit IRBs. These boards agree to conduct an ethical analysis of research for a fee, raising the question of whether economics may influence their decisions.

For-profit IRBs charge fees to review research in a way that complies with federal regulations. Their goal is to make money by providing a service to the research community. In some cases, they conduct reviews for individual researchers who are not affiliated with a particular institution. In others, institutions themselves, in private industry, for example, establish a contract with for-profit IRBs to review their proposals for a year.

Unlike IRBs staffed by volunteers, for-profit IRBs have a direct economic interest in conducting reviews, so the question arises whether they can be as independent. Volunteers can afford to say no to particular research protocols, but a for-profit board would seem to have an interest in keeping clients happy. If the IRB insists on sweeping changes or refuses approval altogether, clients may go elsewhere for approval.

It is fair to ask whether the potential for conflict of interest is just as great in nonprofit IRBs. For example, members of a university board might have a strong interest in maintaining the flow of research money into the university. Even though individual members might not directly profit from the research, this interest could color the way they treat research proposals. Might this be another version of the potential conflict of interest raised about for-profit IRBs? And if so, is it possible to eliminate (or minimize) potential conflicts of interest?

Study Questions

1. What is the key worry about IRBs that make a profit from reviewing research studies?

2. Many universities depend heavily on research funds from government and private agencies. Is it not true that university IRBs also have a set of interests that may color the way in which they review protocols? How, if at all, might volunteer IRBs at universities differ in the way they carry out reviews compared with for-profit IRBs?

4.13

Willowbrook Hepatitis Studies

The name Willowbrook is permanently associated with scandal, mostly because of the way this state school housed severely retarded children. The school is also known for invaluable hepatitis studies conducted there. In fact, these studies established for the first time that two strains of hepatitis existed. Although the value of the studies has never been in question, their methods remain under continuing debate, involving as they did feeding live hepatitis virus to children. The way in which subjects were recruited is also a matter of controversy.

Willowbrook State School was an institution for the retarded on Staten Island, New York. At the time of a 1972 television exposé, it could hold approximately 5,400 inmates and had approximately 1 attendant for every 50 to 60 children. Its inmates were predominantly African-Americans and Puerto Ricans with chronic, incurable, and profound retardation. Many of these children were housed as if in a warehouse and left unclothed and soiled in their own excrement. Many of the forty buildings had no furniture. The 1972 exposé was not the first. In 1965, New York Senator Robert Kennedy called Willowbrook "a reproach to us all . . . we cannot tolerate a new snakepit."

During the 1950s, Dr. Saul Krugman was the director of research at Willowbrook. He knew that many children there would develop hepatitis because of overcrowding. In fact, many members of the staff developed hepatitis as well. Dr. Krugman also knew that the virus responsible for hepatitis did not have hosts outside human beings. He was persuaded that these conditions justified research on the disease in humans. He initiated a project at Willowbrook to study gamma globulin injections to determine whether they would protect the children from infection. The injections did seem to have a strong protective effect.

Dr. Krugman then admitted new residents of the school to special quarters and fed them virus samples he had collected from the other children. By tracking virus exposures and the pattern of symptoms that followed, he was led to the conclusion that hepatitis had two strains, A and B. A had shorter incubation and was highly communicable, whereas B had longer incubation and was less communicable.

When protest arose regarding his exposure of these children to hepatitis virus, Dr. Krugman defended his work. If he had not infected the children as part of research, they would have developed hepatitis anyway because of their school's communal housing. This research, he said, was akin to an experiment in nature, and no level of improved hygiene would have protected the children. He noted, too, that he had been given permission from parents to experiment on their children.

It is true that children were enrolled with parental consent. A letter explaining the research was sent to parents whose children were on a waiting list for admission to Willowbrook. Immediate admission was the reward for parents who signed the letter; parents who did not provide consent were not assured of immediate admission. The letter is reproduced below.

Willowbrook State School

Office of the Director
Staten Island, New York
November 15, 1958

Dear _____ :

We are studying the possibility of preventing epidemics of hepatitis on a new principle. Virus is introduced and gamma globulin given later to some, so that either no attack or only a mild attack of hepatitis is expected to follow. This may give the children immunity against this disease for life. We should like to give your child this new form of prevention with the hope that it will afford protection.

Permission form is enclosed for your consideration. If you wish to have your child given the benefit of this new preventative, will you so signify by signing the form.

Sincerely,

H. H. Berman, MD
Director

Study Questions

1. How did researchers justify exposing children at Willowbrook to hepatitis infection? How persuasive is their position?

2. Does the letter adequately express the nature, risks, and benefits of the study? Might aspects of agreeing to the experiment be viewed as coercive?

3. Even if the risks of this study were adequately disclosed, do you think researchers would have been justified in exposing children to hepatitis infection?

Adapted from David J. Rothman, Sheila M. Rothman, *The Willowbrook Wars* (New York: Harper & Row, 1984).

4.14

Conflict of Interest in HIV-Prevention Studies

Researchers can apply to the federal government for certificates of confidentiality that permit them to observe potentially illegal behavior without having to report crimes or stand liable for failing to do so. These certificates offer exemption from legal responsibilities and liability only when research data cannot be obtained in any other way. Researchers can still face profound ethical conflicts, however, as the hypothetical case below demonstrates.

In the late 1980s, Alfred Walton was finishing a degree in medical anthropology. He was studying drug-use rituals in Seattle to find ways of reducing HIV infection among people who use needles to inject drugs. His goal was to provide a descriptive study of how needles are shared for this purpose. The rituals involved were not well understood at the time. With this description in hand, researchers could identify interventions that would decrease needle sharing or increase the use of clean needles. At the time, the study was of extreme interest for AIDS prevention. Walton applied for and received a certificate of confidentiality for this study.

Part of Walton's task was to win the confidence of Seattle drug users. He assured them that he would not report anyone to legal authorities. After several months, Walton won the confidence of about twenty drug users, and they came to accept his being around, watching them, and taking notes. Gradually, these people told him about their lives and let him watch them inject drugs. In a private conversation, Ray R. told Walton that he had been diagnosed with HIV two years earlier: "It was bad news to hear, but after the life I've had what could I expect?" Walton offered him sympathy, but the two men never returned to the topic again.

One afternoon, while observing three men and two women injecting heroin, Walton saw Ray take the needle from his arm and hand it to the man next to him. The man wiped the exterior of the needle slightly but did not clean the interior. He then filled the syringe with the heroin solution and prepared his arm for injection.

Walton was dumbfounded that Ray would hand a dirty needle to someone without cleaning it. He knew that a certificate of confidentiality covered his research so he was not obliged to report this behavior. Walton also knew that if the second man became HIV-infected he (Walton) could not be sued for failing to disclose. Nevertheless, he wondered if he had an ethical obligation to intervene. If he did, he might lose the confidence of the people he wanted to study, and that could slow the research necessary to help control this infection. He was not there to save anyone from HIV infection, he told himself; he was there only to study the rituals of drug injection.

Study Questions

1. What is the logic of freeing researchers from legal responsibilities to report crime? How important do you believe this exemption is to research of the kind described?

2. Could the information sought in this study been obtained in a way that would not have required a certificate of confidentiality?

3. Despite the certificate of confidentiality, do you believe Walton had an obligation to intervene and find a way to stop the man from injecting a possibly infected needle into his arm? What if his actions in doing so fundamentally compromised the research, destroying the trusting relationship he had with the drug users?

5
Social Effects of Research

Introduction

It is sometimes assumed that all increases in scientific knowledge are to the good. Even the terms we use in discussing scientific outcomes—*advance, progress*—betray an optimism that research is the very instrument of human worth and happiness. To be sure, research *is* essential to the enlargement of human hope and happiness in many ways. This is especially true with regard to lifting the burdens of illness and disease, burdens that all too easily erode meaningful human life. Nevertheless, it does not follow that all research is of equal value or that constraints should not be placed on ways in which it is conducted.

Evaluating the Social Impact of Research
Research has intended and unintended consequences, some of which are far-reaching indeed. For example, the intended consequence of research in infectious disease

might be to identify new methods of prevention. The unintended consequence of successful research is that as infectious diseases are brought under control, people become vulnerable to other conditions such as cancer and heart disease. Part of the task of bioethics is to identify and, to the extent possible, protect against objectionable effects. Research does not occur in a vacuum, and social consequences deserve consideration as do motives and process.

It is true that a great deal of research has been performed without attempts to determine its long-term social effects. Indeed, some of the most important scientific discoveries occurred without anyone conducting what is the equivalent of an ethics impact study. For example, scientists who developed and perfected the combustible engine did not undertake analysis to determine whether, on balance, the engine would be a boon or bane to humanity. Neither did those who harnessed and distributed electricity make their discoveries only after considering ways in which they would transform society. No one argued in advance against the development of engines and electricity on the grounds that they would transform war in swift and terrible ways. No broad public discussion addressed the ethics of developing airplanes, trying to assess the profound implications that this transportation would have on the environment or on the distribution of disease. It goes without saying that the secrecy that surrounded the development of nuclear weapons precluded widespread analysis of their impact.[1]

What mechanisms are in place for evaluating the social impact of research projects? As things stand, IRBs are the front line for identifying and deterring objectionable biomedical research that involves human subjects. As part of their responsibilities, should they also consider long-term effects? In fact, federal regulations specifically bar this function: "The IRB should not consider possible long-range effects of applying knowledge gained in the research (for example, the possible effects of the research on public policy) as among those research risks that fall within the purview of its responsibility."[2] There are many good reasons for this exclusion. As IRBs can have as few as five members, it would be difficult to ask them to sit in judgment on the broad social effects of research. They would ordinarily have neither the time nor the resources to evaluate whether, all things considered, society needs yet another hypertension drug or whether a particular line of xenograft research will be too costly, too unsafe, and too socially disruptive in the long run. Those questions should be discussed and evaluated, but it is asking too much of IRBs to involve them in such an overall social evaluation. The fact is that no single body has the capacity or duty to determine the ultimate desirability of research projects. Neither is there a single body that determines what studies should be implemented quickly and what should be relegated to the back burner. The responsibility for assessing the social effects of research is widely diffused across researchers, government, academic institutions, nongovernment organizations such as advocacy groups and charities, and the public at large.

Evaluating Research and Priorities in a Liberal Democracy

In the United States, both private and public sectors sponsor ambitious research programs. In the private sector, researchers use their own funds to stake out domains of interest and pursue them, typically guided by the goal of commercially valuable products. Indeed, private corporations are one of the main sources of research sponsorship in the world today. The right to conduct research is rooted as a matter of law in the First Amendment right to free speech. Despite this constitutional foundation, researchers must, of course, abide by government regulations that guide research with humans or when bringing drugs and medical devices to market. Otherwise, they have a free hand in what they pursue and how they do so. For example, many jurisdictions have no legal impediments to the production of human embryos for research purposes. If scientists in these jurisdictions want to use their own money to engage in this area of study, they are free to do so.

To say that researchers in the private sphere are free to set their own agendas and conduct research that might not be possible with government money is not to say that they and their sponsoring corporations are blind to ethical issues. Some research firms have ethics advisory groups as a way of addressing concerns about the methods and effects of their projects. One such biotech company is Advanced Cell Technology (ACT), in Massachusetts; it conducts research related to somatic cell nuclear transfer and transgenic animals. The company believes its human cloning research can lead the way to important scientific and therapeutic discoveries. It does maintain an ethics advisory board and in 2002 described its function this way: "The ACT Ethics Advisory Board [EAB] exists to provide independent and informed advice to the leadership of Advanced Cell Technology on matters of ethical importance raised by company activities and research programs. Members of the board are independent scholars or professionals with no financial ties to ACT. As a matter of EAB policy, members receive only a modest fee (set at the equivalent to the National Institutes of Health per diem for grant reviewers) for attendance at each of the Board's quarterly meetings. The EAB serves ACT in an advisory function. As individuals and as a body, EAB members have 'the power of the pen,' permitting them to openly dissent from ACT response to or implementation of EAB recommendations."[3] Indeed, members of some advisory boards disagree with how companies conduct research. Obviously, such dissidents are not likely to remain on advisory boards for very long. It should also be said that the effect of these boards in identifying and deterring research that is objectionable, especially with respect to long-term consequences, is not well studied.

Health advocacy groups are often the source of funds for research, with money raised and applied according to their own interests. Many groups, for example, pursue research and treatment for particular diseases. The magnitude of their effect depends on their fund-raising abilities, not on the relative social importance of the disorder or disease in question. It can often happen that certain diseases do not attract broad funding because they do not affect very many people. This does not mean those diseases are not profoundly disordering; they often are. Some bioethicists contend that certain diseases have a high claim to research priority precisely because they are so disordering, regardless of how many or how few people are affected.[4] Individual parties are free, nonetheless, to spend their money as they see fit, whether their target project improves the quality of life of many people only a little or of just a few people a great deal.

In the public sphere, the government makes money available to researchers through its own institutions or through external grant programs to work in particular areas it deems important in medicine, agriculture, defense, and so on. Legislative choices and the goals of federal agencies often drive government-funded projects. The federal government has instituted advisory commissions to study particular problems and make recommendations about the nature and scope of research projects. During the Clinton administration, the National Bioethics Advisory Commission issued a number of reports on research involving human cloning and human embryonic stem cells.[5] George W. Bush's President's Council on Bioethics issued its own recommendations about research involving cloning of human beings.[6] Final decisions about whether to act on these recommendations rest, of course, with legislatures and federal agencies.

Consequences of Genetic Research

One project is worth mentioning in detail because of its companion social effects program, a very visible example of an attempt to discern and prepare for the effects of research. Beginning in 1990, an international coalition of researchers in the United States, United Kingdom, Japan, and elsewhere undertook the Human Genome Project (HGP).[7] This project has completed a working map and sequencing of the human genome and the genome of several other organisms.

Many people have expressed concern that genetic tests made possible by the HGP will be used prejudicially in employment and insurance, excluding people with genetic disorders and those at risk of developing such disorders in the future. One author pointed to the way in which certain burdens of genetic testing fall on women facing reproductive choices.[8] Others predicted a profound gap between being able to test for a genetic disorder and being able to do anything about it. An important danger is that genetics will be treated in a reductive way: treating complex phenomena as if they were reducible to a particular genetic trait.[9] Genetic research will also open new possibilities for banking and using biological samples for commercial purposes, raising questions about who is entitled to what in such cases.[10]

To assuage certain social worries, the sponsors of the HGP set aside a portion of the total budget to assess ethical, legal, and social implications (ELSI). The goals of this program have varied over time, but as of 2003 the program focuses on the following issues: "1. *Privacy and Fairness in the Use and Interpretation of Genetic Information*. Activities in this area examine the meaning of genetic information and how to prevent its misinterpretation or misuse. 2. *Clinical Integration of New Ge-*

netic Technologies. These activities examine the impact of genetic testing on individuals, families and society, and inform clinical policies related to genetic testing and counseling. 3. *Issues Surrounding Genetics Research.* Activities in this area focus on informed consent and other research-ethics review issues related to the design, conduct, participation in and reporting of genetics research. 4. *Public and Professional Education.* This area includes activities that provide education on genetics and related ELSI issues to health professionals, policy makers and the general public."[11]

Projects such as this involve public education, draft recommendations to protect against the worst effects of genetic testing, historical analysis of projects, and so on. The ELSI program set a precedent for ways to think about the social consequences of research. By the same token, this set-aside is itself something worth analysis. Did simultaneous and anticipatory analysis help guide actual policy and prevent objectionable misuses of genetic research? Or was it simply a full-employment act for bioethics, as some critics seemed to think? It remains to be seen how widely ELSI-style research will be adopted for other major research initiatives. (Further discussion of ethical issues in genetic research may be found in the introduction to chapter 7.)

Consultation and Transparency

No one can predict all the ways in which research may transform society. It is impossible to prepare for all possible outcomes, but a useful starting point is to extend the paramount dictum of medicine to all research: first, do no harm. One way to help ensure that no harm is done by way of creating or deepening social disadvantages, is to involve the people most likely to be affected in dialogue or consultation. Toward this end, some bioethicists have proposed a principle of community consent.[12]

According to the principle of community consent, researchers would be obliged to ask communities for degrees of permission to conduct various kinds of research. This proposal is problematic in a number of ways. What counts, first of all, as a community affected by research? Suppose a researcher wishes to study homosexuality or a particular genetic trait associated with obese women. Who counts as "community" in these instances? Homosexuality occurs across all age, cultural, and ethnic groups, as does obesity. Who would count as the "consentor" in these instances? To get past such difficulties, researchers now accept the notion of community consultation. The community under study may be approached through its institutions— tribal councils, schools, religious groups, and so on—to advise on the nature and meaning of research. In this manner researchers hope to advise and engage subjects in a way that respects them but does not raise difficult questions about who is entitled to consent on behalf of a community as a whole.

In addition to this kind of consultation, it is ethically advisable that research be transparent. Where there is uncertainty, there will be speculation. And uncertainties about the nature and scope of research will invite speculation of all kinds. While it is important to recognize the importance of protecting commercial aspects of private research, researchers nevertheless should try to explain their goals and methods to the public in an accessible way. Indeed, transparency can help promote public discussion that is essential to informed decision making at the political level.

In many cases, analysis of the social value of research will occur after the fact. Scientific projects sometimes outstrip even the most far-seeing expectations. When this happens—when research outcomes alter the status quo with regard to access and equity to social goods—it remains important that all the tools of democracy be deployed: deliberation, education, and public discussion. To paraphrase Socrates, an unexamined community life is not worth living.

References

1. Richard Rhodes, *Dark Sun: The Making of the Hydrogen Bomb* (New York: Simon and Schuster, 1995).

2. 45 C.F.R. 46.111.

3. Downloaded from www.advancedcell.com September 9, 2002.

4. Leonard M. Fleck, "Just Genetics: A Problem Agenda," in Timothy F. Murphy, Marc A. Lappé, eds., *Justice and the Human Genome Project* (Berkeley: University of California Press, 1994), pp. 133–152.

5. Robert Cook Deegan, *The Gene Wars: Science, Politics, and the Human Genome Project* (New York: W.W. Norton, 1994).

5. National Bioethics Advisory Commission, *Cloning Human Beings* (Washington, DC: NBAC, 1997); and *Issues in Human Stem Cell Research* (Washington, DC: NBAC, 1999).

6. President's Council on Bioethics, *Human Cloning and Human Dignity: An Ethical Inquiry* (Washington, DC: President's Council on Bioethics, 2002).

7. Robert Cook Deegan, *The Gene Wars: Science, Politics, and the Human Genome Project* (New York: W.W. Norton, 1994).

8. Barbara Katz Rothman, *The Book of Life: A Personal Guide to Race, Normality, and the Implications of the Human Genome Project* (Boston: Beacon Press, 2001).

9. Jonathan Michael Kaplan, *The Limits and Lies of Human Genetic Research: Dangers for Social Policy* (New York: Routledge, 2000).

10. Timothy A. Caufield, Bryn Williams-Jones, eds., *The Commercialization of Genetic Research: Legal, Ethical, and Policy Issues* (Dordrecht: Kluwer Academic, 1999).

11. Downloaded from http://www.genome.gov September 9, 2002.

12. Charles Weijer, "Protecting Communities in Research: Philosophical and Pragmatic Challenges," *Cambridge Quarterly of Healthcare Ethics* 1999 (8): 501–513.

5.1

Cloning for Longer Life

Since somatic cell nuclear transfer allows cloning of mammals, the question of cloned human beings has taken on new urgency. A great deal of commentary focused on potential harm to children who might be born through this technology, with emphasis on physical as well as psychological harm. Regardless, cloning may open the way to a mechanism for extending human life, provided those human lives originate through somatic cell nuclear transfer.

Dolly, the sheep born in 1997 through a cloning technique perfected by Ian Wilmut and his colleagues in Scotland, looked like any other Finn Dorset lamb at birth, but questions about her actual age soon arose. Wilmut took the nucleus of an adult sheep's mammary tissue and transferred it, after certain treatment, into an enucleated sheep ovum, a technique called somatic cell nuclear transfer. The resulting cell developed as an embryo, and the developing embryo was transferred into a sheep uterus, where it successfully gestated until birth. Many attempts had failed before this success.

Because the nucleus from the donor somatic cell is the product of a long line of cell division, it has characteristic telomere shortening. Telomeres are DNA patterns that affect the number of times a cell can divide. As cells divide, they typically lose part of the telomere. This fact would predict that Dolly's cells were less capable of new divisions, and she would thus be genetically older than her chronological age. A 1998 study seemed to show that the sheep was in fact older, as far as her telomeres were concerned, than her actual years.

In 2000, a biotechnology company in Massachusetts showed that this effect could be controlled. Researchers at Advanced Cell Technology grew calf cells in culture until they had cycled through about 95 percent of their lifespan as far as their telomeres were concerned. Nuclei from these cells were then transferred into enucleated eggs. In the resultant cloned calves, not only were the telomeres no shorter than those in control animals, they were actually longer; they showed the potential for ninety-three divisions, compared with only sixty-one divisions for cells from animals that had not been cloned. The researchers speculated that this potential might increase the life of the animals by as much as 50 percent. Some were quick to point out that if this were done in humans, people might live as long as 180 to 200 years. It turns out that cloning might prove a key mechanism for extending human life.

Study Questions

1. Do you think that extending human life is a good enough reason to employ somatic cell nuclear transfer to produce human beings?

2. In general, why do you think it would be desirable to extend (or not extend) human life to as much as 200 years of age? What benefits would occur if this were possible? What social harms?

3. Even if it were not desirable to extend human life, can you think of any reason to lengthen lives of other animals?

Adapted from Potter Wickware, "The Science of Cloning," in Glenn McGee, ed., *The Human Cloning Debate,* 2nd ed. (Berkeley, CA: Berkeley Hills Books, 2000), pp. 16–41.

5.2

Sexual Orientation Research

A number of researchers have reported certain biological correlations of sexual orientation. These correlations are links between biological traits and sexual orientation, but their causal relationship, if any, to sexual orientation is unknown. In 1991 a neuroanatomical researcher reported that homosexual men were more likely than heterosexual men to have a smaller neurological structure in the portion of the brain that influences sexual desire. Later, a research team at the National Institutes of Health reported that a section of the X chromosome is shared more commonly by gay male siblings than by straight male siblings. In the context of the social treatment of men and women with homosexual orientation, debate centers on whether this research should be done at all. Some fear that it might profoundly damage the lives of gay men and lesbians. It might be used to identify and eliminate fetuses destined to become homosexual adults, to produce therapy for homosexual orientation, or to extend discrimination in employment and other areas.

In 1984, German sexologist Gunter Schmidt said, "As long as society has not made peace with the homosexuals, research into the possible causes [of homosexuality is] . . . potentially a public danger to . . . [lesbians and gay men]. Seen in this light, it is good that we know so little about what causes heterosexuality and homosexuality." A University of California professor of English, Leo Bersani, thinks that biological research will make it easier for society to identify homosexuals. He worries that the nineteenth-century project of curing homosexuals may succeed beyond its wildest dreams if determinants of sexual orientation are identified—science may be used in "gender cleansing."

German philosopher Udo Schüklenk said that sexual orientation research should be halted in all societies that discriminate against lesbians and gay men. It is feared that dictatorships and other autocratic governments would love to be able to use scientific methods to identify and eliminate homosexual people. In a letter to the editor of *Science,* United States biologists Anne Fausto-Sterling and Evan Balaban claimed that "the scientific debate about the origins of homosexuality is taking place in the midst of a highly political one about the place of gay men and lesbians in our social fabric. Given the increased frequency of hate crimes directed against homosexuals, it is fair and literal to say that lives are at stake." Many individuals also worried about "search and destroy" prenatal diagnostic tests. In 1994, philosopher Frederick Suppe argued that this research is not only potentially stigmatizing but that it is also scientifically uninteresting because it opens up no new interesting domain of inquiry. He therefore counseled that it be abandoned.

By contrast, Timothy F. Murphy, professor of bioethics at the University of Illinois College of Medicine at Chicago, considered that it is probably not possible to prohibit this research because scientists may act on their own, and because genetic or neurological contributions to sexual orientation will probably be discovered in the fullness of time anyway. He claimed that the most important question is not whether the research is conducted, but whether society has mechanisms in place to protect gay men and lesbians from its discriminatory applications.

Study Questions

1. How persuasive is the idea that identifying the origins of homosexuality is an important goal? In what way is it important to have this knowledge?

2. What possible effects might this research have, and would prohibition against it be the only way to deal with objectionable effects?

3. How convincing is the view that sexual orientation research will actually improve the social status of homosexual men and women because it will dispel myths, given the fact that there is no adequate scientific account of sexual orientation?

Adapted from Timothy F. Murphy, *Gay Science: The Ethics of Sexual Orientation Research* (New York: Columbia University Press, 1997), p. 55; and Anne Fausto-Sterling, Evan Balaban, "Genetics and Male Sexual Orientation," *Science* 1993 (261) 5126:1259.

5.3

Genetic Research and Forced Choices

Using standpoint theory, some feminist analysis looks at genetic research in terms of the impact it has across various populations, often women, children, and the poor. In the cases below, the impact—and therefore the ethics—of genetic research are evaluated in terms of access to reproductive choices. Development of genetic interventions raises important questions of social justice.

Case 1: "Maria and Reinaldo Sanchez, twenty-seven and thirty years old, arrived in Brooklyn, New York, from Puerto Rico, with their four school-age children. Although they knew little English, both got jobs in a restaurant, earning minimum wages. Within a month, Maria discovered she was pregnant. After a routine triple screen, she was advised to see a genetic counselor and undergo chorionic villus sampling or amniocentesis. Most of her visits to the prenatal clinic were delayed by her inability to secure appointments that did not conflict with her child care and job responsibilities, and by the unavailability of a Spanish interpreter. By the time Maria was told that her fetus had Down syndrome, she was twenty weeks pregnant. The clinic did not provide second-trimester terminations, but she was given the name of a clinic in another city where she might obtain the procedure. Maria called the clinic and was told that a second-trimester abortion would cost considerably more than she could afford."

Case 2. "Sonya and Rob Smith, both thirty-six years old, had two children, ages six and two. Rob was a community obstetrician with a successful practice. Sonya was a full-time homemaker. Their young child, Alex, had problems learning to walk and appeared delayed in his speech development. At a routine visit to the pediatrician with both children, Sonya expressed her concern about Alex's slow development. The pediatrician suggested consultation with a geneticist. When Sonya called the genetics center, she was asked if she would like both children to be fully evaluated. She was also asked to have her pediatrician send complete copies of both children's medical records to the clinic. During their appointment, attended by both parents, extensive family histories were taken and physician exams performed on both children. A 'routine' set of genetic tests was ordered for Alex, and the result indicated that he had fragile X syndrome. His sister was tested next and found not to be a carrier for the condition. Follow-up counseling prompted Sonya to contact various relatives and alert them to the risk of fragile X syndrome in family members. The Smiths' insurance plan covered all appointments and all of the recommended testing."

Study Questions

1. What disadvantages do the Sanchezes face in making choices about having and not having children? To what extent do you think that society is responsible for their difficulties? What advantages do the Smiths have when making choices about having and not having children? To what extent do you think that society is responsible for their advantages?

2. To what extent is it proper to conduct research in genetics when large segments of the population will not benefit? Is continued investment in genetic research justified when advances might come at the expense of people with nothing to gain from that research?

3. How well does feminist methodology work in terms of using standpoint theory to illuminate relevant ethical aspects of resource allocation and research priorities?

From Mary Briody Mahowald, *Genes, Women, Equality* (New York: Oxford University Press, 2000), p. 99.

5.4

Earth's Population

Doomsday prophets often point to the growing size of Earth's population and predict a dire fate as a result. In 1679, Antoni van Leeuwenhoek estimated that our planet could support 13.4 billion people. That figure has been scaled up and down since that time, as analysts debate ways of producing a meaningful estimate, with some holding that no meaningful, long-term estimate can be given. Nevertheless, the size of the human population remains a matter of ethical concern, especially with regard to research designed to supply the resources essential to life. The question is whether ethical considerations about population size ought to play a role in how research is conducted.

The number of people Earth can sustain depends on a variety of factors. In any calculation, one must consider what level of material well-being is desirable. After all, many more people could be sustained at very low levels than at higher levels. The technological skills and capacity of a society would also factor into the matter. For example, if crops could be modified through genetic interventions to produce greater food yields, this would uphold greater and greater numbers of people. It is an open question, however, whether technological advances capable of maintaining an increasingly large population can be guaranteed.

Some political systems are much more conducive to increases in population than others. The nature of political and social arrangements also bears on the ability to feed, clothe, house, and offer health care to a population. Distribution systems in knowledge and material goods are just as important as food and housing.

Population size would also depend on the control societies gain over natural phenomena such as floods, volcanic eruptions, and other disasters. If these could be predicted and controlled, the population could increase. Another factor concerns the kinds of families people see as desirable. People might believe that they should contribute to the world no more than a single replacement for themselves. In this case, issues related to quality of life, and not technology, would dictate population size.

Despite the importance of population, questions about the ethics of interventions that will increase Earth's capacity to sustain more human beings are rarely raised. Perhaps that is because they tend to be eclipsed by short-term needs.

Study Questions

1. Depending on what is desired for the population, Earth could probably sustain many more human beings than it already does. Are there any reasons to think that there should be more humans—maybe many times more—than already exist?

2. What reasons are there to reduce the total number of humans on the planet? What domains of research would be especially important if this were to be achieved?

Adapted from Joel E. Cohen, "How Many People Can the Earth Support?" in Dan E. Beauchamp, Bonnie Steinbock, eds., *New Ethics for the Public's Health* (New York: Oxford University Press, 1999), pp. 330–338.

Heart Transplants: Racial Politics

Scientific experiments are influenced by the social milieu, and this was true for heart transplantations. The following case raises important questions about subject selection in a country that, at the time of the transplant, formally set races apart as a matter of law and privilege. In such a setting, it is well worth considering what sorts of people ought to be chosen as the first to undergo major innovations such as heart transplantations.

South African physician Christian Barnaard said his hospital advised him that the first recipient of an experimental heart transplant should be a white patient, otherwise nonwhite parties might accuse him of exploiting nonwhites. The same worry extended to the heart donor if the heart to be transplanted came from a nonwhite.

In 1967, when he was prepared to undertake the procedure and the first heart became available, Barnaard asked if the woman donor was colored, a term referring to black-skinned Africans. He feared that if she was, her heart could not be used. She was not, and he performed the surgery.

This sensitivity to race was not just a concern of the physicians involved: many journalists covering the story asked if the donor was white. At that time, the race of blood donors was recorded, and recipients of blood were allowed to choose the race of donors. However, transracial transplantation of kidneys had already been performed in South Africa. Despite sensitivity to the question, race did not emerge as a major social concern in heart transplantation. By and large, most whites, blacks, and ethnic Indians did not worry about donating or receiving transplantations from other groups.

Study Questions

1. This case shows the way in which social sensitivities can influence the way in which research is conducted. Do you think an injustice was committed in making a decision that the first donor and recipient of a transplanted heart could only be white?

2. In the United States, a very small number of organ donors have tried to restrict transplantation of their organs to members of their own race. This is sometimes called "directed donation," but no organ-procurement organization honors such requests. Do you think such restrictions are morally defensible?

Adapted from Gregory E. Pence, *Classical Cases in Medical Ethics* (New York: McGraw-Hill, 1990), pp. 292, 322.

5.6

Contracts with Research Subjects

The subject of treating research subjects equitably has received a lot of attention. The case below involves a written contract that would carry punitive fines if its terms were violated. Alan F. Benjamin agreed to this contract so as not to assert privilege over the concerns of the community. In a practical way, the contract addresses the fact that ethnographers are not always sensitive to the needs of the community. In the end, it gave the subjects a say in how they were represented. It is worth discussing whether such a contract is morally desirable or whether it could significantly compromise research interests.

In 1991 Alan F. Benjamin went to Curaçao in the Netherland Antilles to conduct a study of the ethnic identity of a religious congregation. That group, the United Netherlands Portuguese Congregation Mikva Israel-Emanuel, dates from 1651. Given its long history, Benjamin wanted to assess the many changes the group has undergone. He intended his work to be the basis of a doctoral dissertation and for other publications. As a small group on a small island, members of the congregation worried about public opinion if the research put them in a bad light. Before beginning his study, Benjamin negotiated with the group and signed a contract regarding how his findings would be reported.

Specifically, the contract stipulated that a review committee of the congregation could approve all publications that dealt with them and would reject only material that they thought would have an adverse effect on their reputation. Benjamin agreed that the congregation was in a better position to evaluate whether and what information would adversely effect their reputation. On the other hand, the congregation conceded that Benjamin was in a better position to evaluate what findings and interpretations would be significant and therefore worth publishing. Benjamin agreed that he would use only data that were verified as correct by the committee. The review committee could not, however, withhold approval from interpretations and conclusions drawn from this factual information, as long as the congregation's reputation did not suffer. Benjamin agreed to submit drafts of publications to the committee, with a few exceptions. He would not submit term papers, proposals, or dissertation drafts as long as these materials went before academic scholars only and carried the instruction "for your eyes only." The final draft of the dissertation would, however, have to receive approval from the committee.

If any violation of this process occurred, Benjamin agreed to pay to the congregation a fine of 5,000 Netherland Antilles francs (approximately $2,500 at the time) per day. The fine would accrue from the date of publication of the unapproved material to the day on which all copies of the material were withdrawn.

Study Questions

1. What are the chief benefits of involving members of the study in this way? Are there benefits to the researcher? To community members? To the study itself?

2. Do you think obstacles to an accurate study of this group could arise through the group's veto power over some data?

3. To what extent do you think this contractual relationship should serve as a model for all social science research on populations, particularly small and socially vulnerable ones?

Adapted from Alan F. Benjamin, "Contracts and Covenant in Curaçao: Reciprocal Relationships in Scholarly Research," in Nancy M. P. King, Gail A. Henderson, Jane Stein, eds., *Beyond Regulation: Ethics in Human Subject Research* (Chapel Hill: University of North Carolina Press, 1999), pp. 49–66.

5.7

Compensation for Research Injuries

At the present time, no federal requirement or social consensus requires researchers to pay the costs of injuries sustained in the course of research. For example, a subject enrolled in a drug trial may develop a severe immune reaction or suffer liver-related problems. Researchers may treat any immediate symptoms, especially if they are life-threatening, but they are not required to pay long-term costs of adverse effects. The process of informed consent is considered sufficient to advise subjects about this risk, and ethics committees rarely stand in the way of this arrangement. However, this approach has its critics.

Federal regulations are clear that, when risk is greater than minimal, researchers must advise potential subjects whether compensation will be available for injuries and adverse events sustained in the course of a study. They must, for example, advise what treatments are available, what they consist of, and how further information about this aspect of the research may be obtained. However, it is not required that researchers provide such medical care.

A number of bioethics commissions have recommended finding a way to provide the required care. For example, in 1982, the President's Commission for the Study of Ethical Problems in Medicine and Biomedical and Behavioral Research recommended that the federal government initiate efforts to implement and evaluate possible methods of compensation. In 2001, the National Bioethics Advisory Commission called on the government to study the need for a compensation program.

Stephen Guest indicated that research subjects are used primarily for the benefit of others. Therefore they should be paid for injuries they sustain in the course of the research, a state of affairs that is not now widely accepted. Guest did not believe that all injuries should be compensated, because some are very minor, and people should be asked to waive compensation for those. Nevertheless, if subjects are seriously injured, they often have little recourse. They might sue, but this puts a great deal of burden on an already injured party.

Some organizations, such as the British Pharmaceutical Industry, recommend adoption of a no-fault policy of compensation for healthy subjects. That is, in case of injury, a subject must simply show that the research was the cause, not that negligence was involved. Once this causal relationship was determined, researchers would be obliged to cover the costs. If patients are involved as subjects, the British Pharmaceutical Industry also advises no-fault compensation for serious injury "of an enduring and disabling character (including exacerbation of an existing condition) and not for temporary pain or discomfort or less serious or curable complaints." Guest stated that Local Research Ethics Committees should withhold approval from all research protocols that do not offer such protections to subjects in experiments involving more than negligible risk.

Study Questions

1. At the present time, researchers may assume responsibility to treat immediate consequences of a research intervention. For example, if a patient had a seizure in reaction to an experimental drug, researchers would ordinarily assume responsibility for its immediate treatment. However, they do not normally assume responsibility for long-term consequences, such as brain damage that developed as a result of the seizures. Those costs would be borne by the subject. The proposal to compensate research subjects for injury is, therefore, far reaching. What is the main reason for changing the status quo and shifting the cost of research-related injuries to researchers rather than subjects?

2. Suppose a subject in a study examining the effect of psychological disorders on sleep experiences panic attacks during the study. He worries that the researchers will mistreat him while he is asleep and exhibits profound anxiety. Suppose that he claimed that it was research that worsened his anxiety and that therefore he should be compensated for treatment he requires. Do you think that difficulties distinguishing injury from preexisting conditions or problems unrelated to the study would make it impossible to design a compensation program for research injuries?

Adapted from Stephen Guest, "Compensation for Subjects of Medical Research: The Moral Rights of Patients and the Power of Research Ethics Committees," *Journal of Medical Ethics* 1997 (23): 181–185. For further information on research-related injury, see Robert Levine, *Ethics and Regulation of Clinical Research* (Baltimore: Urban & Schwarzenberg, 1986), chapter 6.

5.8
___

Nude Posture Photographs

The invention of the camera provoked a variety of innovative medical uses. In the case below, what began as a benign intervention to identify spine problems blossomed into a full-scale eugenics study intent on linking posture with character traits and intelligence.

Until the 1960s, many colleges routinely took "physique photographs." These were used to identify difficulties with posture, and students with problems were sometimes sent to posture classes. The photographs were taken at some of the most prestigious schools in the nation: Yale, Smith, Vassar, Mt. Holyoke, University of California, University of Pennsylvania, and many more. Researchers occasionally took comparable photographs at such places as the Oregon Hospital for the Criminally Insane. Students were typically photographed in the nude, from the front, side, and back, with metal pins positioned along their spines that pointed to problems in posture. The photographs were identified by date, name or initials of subject, age, height, and weight.

One of the leading proponents of these photographs was W. H. Sheldon, who together with E. A. Hooton, led the Institute for Physique Studies at Columbia University. These men took advantage of the tradition of the physique photograph and tried to persuade other institutions to give them access to photographs. Their interest went beyond posture. Based on their interpretation of the physique, they believed that they could assign a three-digit number that represented the individual's character. This interpretation was based on a theory of three basic body types they thought were correlated with people's capacities: ectomorph (slim), mesomorph (ideal), and endomorph (round). The researchers believed it was possible to predict the character of the person from body type and to predict the nature of his or her social contributions. Professor Sheldon presented his analyses in a book entitled *Atlas of Man*; he never finished a planned companion volume on women.

Many subjects for this study were never aware that their photographs were used for research. They believed that the pictures were routine and that they were for their stated purpose: evaluation of posture. Between 1956 and the 1970s, some colleges began to take steps to destroy these photographs. Alumni were outraged at the way in which these photographs were used. Nevertheless, some of these photographs still exist, although most appear to be held in archives that limit access and use.

Study Questions

1. Do you think it would be possible to maintain that no consent was necessary for this study since the photographed persons would not be identified?

2. In what sense, if any, were subjects of this study harmed?

3. Would it be important to keep the photographs that remain as part of the historical record of research in the United States, or is there a convincing argument that all these photographs should be destroyed?

Adapted from Ron Rosenblaum, "The Great Ivy League Nude Posture Photo Scandal," *New York Times Magazine,* Jan. 15, 1995, pp. 26–31, 40, 46, 55–56.

5.9

Disclosure of Study Results

Protecting confidentiality in research can work against the interests of subjects, if researchers withhold information that might be useful to them. The hypothetical case below raises questions of whether a study agreement should be breached after the subject has waived all right to see the results.

Angus Davidson, age forty-two, reads in the local newspaper that the university medical center in his city has concluded a ten-year study on cancer recurrence. According to the article, the study showed that patients with a particular biological marker are much more likely to have a recurrence of cancer after surgery than those without it.

Doctors at that center removed a tumor from Davidson three years earlier, and he recalls signing a form giving permission to use his tissue in research, although no particular study was identified. He contacts the investigator named in the newspaper, Dr. Richard Schone, saying he would like to know whether his tissue was used and, if so, whether he has the biological marker. Davidson says that if he has the marker, he will cash in his retirement funds and travel the world. If he is in the low-risk group, he will continue working and count on having a long life. Schone tells Davidson that he will call him back after reviewing the records.

Reviewing those records, Schone finds Davidson's consent form, the code to the tissue records, and coded reports on all tissue samples in the study. The consent form indicated that any information about tissue samples would be connected to medical records by a number known only to the immediate research team.

Schone is unsure what to do next. Over and above the question of whether he has an obligation to tell Davidson about his test result, he is worried that Davidson might not appreciate the nature of the study. The results were important, but they are not precise enough to counsel individuals about their exact risk of cancer recurrence. Schone is also concerned that he is not Davidson's regular physician and does not want to assume responsibility for his care. Indeed, because of his research involvement it has been many years since he dealt with patients directly.

Yet Schone has told Davidson that he will call. Schone wonders whether he should use the code to see whether Davidson's tissue marker put him in the high-risk group. If so, what should he tell him?

Study Questions

1. It is possible to learn whether or not Mr. Davidson has the specific marker that predicts recurrence of his cancer. Do you believe that this information is, in fact, useful for people to have? Is there any reason for withholding predictions about future disease from people?

2. How valid is Dr. Schone's worry that he might have to enter into a physician-patient relationship with Mr. Davidson if he decides to pass the information along to him? Do you think that this concern is reason enough not to give Mr. Davidson the information?

3. If Dr. Schone makes an exception for Mr. Davidson, do you think he would have an ethical obligation to disclose to all subjects the results of the study whether or not they have the biological marker?

Prepared by Robert Folberg, Frances B. Geever Professor, Department of Pathology, University of Illinois College of Medicine at Chicago.

5.10

Research Funded by Taxpayers

Does the public have a claim to inventions funded by the government? It might seem fair to require that inventions funded through taxes become the property of the public. This is not the case, however, as the government has adopted a policy intended to bring the greatest number of inventions to market in the fastest way possible. The logic of this is stated in the case below. It is possible to object to this view in whole or in part. The more stringent objection is that products developed with government money should belong to the public as a matter of public domain. The less stringent objection is that whereas profit to the inventors spurs creativity and productivity, an amount of the profits should go to the public, for example, to fund additional research or direct medical care.

The United States federal government is one of the largest funders of research involving drugs and medical devices; however, it does not usually assume patent rights to inventions made with this money. It is committed to the view that individual initiative is better for bringing such products to market than it would be. Therefore, law and policy let individuals who use federal money for innovations profit without requiring monies returned to the government. If individual researchers could not profit or stood to profit less, according to this view, they would be less innovative and less committed to improved medical treatments. The government does retain "marching-in" rights. If government agencies decide that an inventor is not doing enough to bring a new, federally funded product to market, they can intervene and assume control over the product. In the main, however, official policy is to fund researchers and leave the process of marketing to them.

Critics propose that the consumer is thus forced to pay twice for new health interventions: once with taxes, and a second time by purchasing the drug or device at whatever cost the maker thinks the market will bear. They insist that costs of such new products could be kept considerably lower if the government put the results of federally sponsored research into the public domain, where anyone could have access to the information.

Study Questions

1. What incentives do researchers have to apply for money from the federal government to create new medical drugs and devices?

2. Why does government policy give researchers the right to patent, produce, and license drugs and devices they develop even though these innovations were developed with taxpayer money?

3. Do you think that the criticism that users of medical devices and drugs pay twice is fair? Is it possible to imagine a system that rewards innovation but also works to keep the cost of new drugs and devices low?

For further information see Timothy F. Murphy, "Ethical Aspects of the Human Genome Project," in Peter Singer, Helga Kuhse, eds., *Companion to Bioethics* (Oxford: Blackwell Press, 1998), pp. 198–205.

Priorities in Health Care: The Aged and Their Diseases

Given the extent to which health care resources are used extensively in the last years of human life, providing public health care for the elderly has met with political resistance. Critics object to subsidies for elder health care not only because they transfer money from one group to another but because they are not socially efficient. That is, this use of money does not serve the greatest social good. The discussion below argues that money should be spent not simply to help the elderly but to maximize the amount of healthy life possible across society as a whole. It follows from this view that the elderly should receive less research priority in health care than younger groups.

At present, a disproportionate investment goes to medical research of diseases that affect the old. In fact, this research is of marginal benefit in extending life. Eliminating one disease among the elderly will only open up more opportunities for other diseases to occur. For example, controlling heart disease may make cancer more common.

Therefore, it is likely, although not certain, that medical research of primary benefit to the elderly is a poor investment compared with research that primarily benefits the middle-aged. For example, suppose society could invest the same amount of money in a treatment that benefits people in group A (those age eighty to eighty-five years) rather than in group B (those age sixty to eighty years). If the treatment has an equal degree of success in both groups, less social gain is achieved in treating group A than group B. People in group A would benefit for only a few more years, whereas those in group B would benefit for a longer period of time and gain as many as fifteen additional years of life. There would also be less social grief for people who died at an old age than a younger age.

Failing to give priority to life-threatening diseases of the young is an inefficient use of research. The only exceptions would be if research for the elderly produced great savings of life compared with the expenditure, and if older people were seriously shortchanged in another way that their taxes support.

One implication of this position is that more money should be spent on the prevention and treatment of mental illness than physical illness. Mental illness produces disability across the lifespan. Removing this disability would help keep workers productive, whereas lengthening life by adding years toward the end of life would not. With more productive workers, the ratio of dependent-to-productive workers is lower, and this is a net social gain. Therefore the old ought to support reallocation of research away from physical illness to research into mental illness.

Study Questions

1. How convincing is the theory that research money should be spent in a way that extends life years as much as possible rather than on diseases and disorders near the end of life?

2. Would the elderly be treated unjustly if, in fact, less research was devoted to treatments for people in their eighties and nineties?

3. How convincing is the notion that research money should be devoted to mental illness in younger persons rather than diseases of the elderly?

Adapted from Richard Posner, *Aging and Old Age* (Chicago: University of Chicago Press, 1995), pp. 269–273.

Curbing the Methuselah Vote

It is universally agreed that extending human life would have considerable social consequences. The case below raises interesting questions about what this would mean for the democratic process. Should an attempt be made to structure voting by demographic groups to limit undue influence by the very elderly?

The *Chicago Sun-Times-Tribune, Oct. 20, 2020:* President Russell Feingold will address 1,000 delegates today at the opening session of a week-long White House conference on Reforming the American Electoral Process. Delegates will debate whether a fundamental principle of the American political system—one person, one vote—should be reformed to prevent elderly citizens from dominating the political system in the future.

The roots of this debate lie in the development of antiglucose, the inexpensive drug that maintains youthfulness in human body tissues by causing cells to make fewer free radicals, a damaging byproduct of glucose metabolism that ordinarily leads to aging. Widespread consumption of antiglucose by Baby Boomers since it reached the market in 2013 has led the U.S. Bureau of the Census to estimate that people age seventy and older will make up more than half the American electorate by midcentury. By 2080 that group will account for more than 80 percent of the voting population. These estimates have fueled much concern that the United States will become a gerontocracy, with virtually all government expenditures devoted to Social Security, Medicare, and other benefit programs for old people.

The agenda for this week's conference promises that deliberations will be politically explosive. A report developed by one conference planning committee recommends that the U.S. Constitution be amended to disenfranchise citizens when they reach the age of seventy (the age of eligibility for Social Security benefits that will become effective in 2025).

Another committee recommends that with each succeeding decade of life past age sixty, a voter's ballot would not be counted as heavily as those of younger voters. Under this plan, persons aged eighteen to sixty-nine would have one vote, persons age seventy to seventy-nine would have one-half a vote, those age eighty to eighty-nine would have one-quarter, those age ninety to ninety-nine would have one-eighth, and so on until the ballot of a person age 120 to 129 would count as one-sixty-fourth of a vote.

President Feingold has been widely hailed for convening a conference to deal with such a controversial topic.

Study Questions

1. A shift toward longer life—people routinely living into their 120s—would certainly shift political power. What are possible benefits of giving power to the oldest members in a society with very long lives? What are the detriments?

2. What kind of social decision making would be desirable in a society of individuals with radically long lives? For example, should decisions about antiglucose therapy be left to the marketplace: those who want it and can afford it get it? Or should society intervene in ways that offer antiglucose to all persons (or, for that matter, to no persons)? How would you want to see something on this scale of importance decided?

Prepared by Robert H. Binstock, Case Western Reserve University, Cleveland, OH. Presented at the University of Illinois Science, Technology, and Society conference, "The Rejuvenator: Technology and the Transformation of Senescence," October 2000.

The End of a Marriage

Scientists are giving hints about how human life might be extended by protecting it from senescence; however, the effects would have far-reaching consequences. In the case below, the meaning of life extension for marriage is considered. Long marriage is held out as a cultural ideal, but would the extension of human life work to undercut that ideal? Should people avoid making life-long marriage commitments? Perhaps very old people of the future could make marriage contracts for periods of time—ten years or twenty—rather than for a lifetime. If people wanted to remain in relationships, they could renew their contracts; otherwise, their marriages would be dissolved.

The *Chicago Tribune, Oct. 20, 2092:* Sentencing is set for tomorrow in Judge McLean's court in the case of Adam Smythe. Smythe, 138, was convicted in July of murdering his wife of 114 years, Irene. The facts of the case were never in dispute. In a fit of rage, Smythe shot his wife six times, killing her instantly. He willingly confessed to the murder, explaining that she had continued to leave puddles of water about the bathroom sink and countertop, despite his repeated protests over decades.

Smythe and his wife were among the first beneficiaries of the Fountain of Youth genetic therapy first offered to the public in 2018. His lawyers, unable to contest the facts of the murder, focused their defense on the unanticipated outcomes of the treatment, arguing that 114 years of marriage was a duration far beyond what the Smythes had imagined when they married in 1978. It was, they insisted, unreasonable to expect couples to live together for more than a hundred years without serious rancor. The district attorney pointed out that divorce was a legal option, but the defense stated that the Smythes' religion excluded divorce. The jury was apparently unswayed by this defense, as it returned a guilty verdict.

Judge McLean faces difficult choices. Statutes dictate either the death penalty or life in prison without parole. In this case, however, it is not at all clear what a life sentence would mean. In addition, Smythe, in an unusual presentencing move, expressed to the judge his preference for the death penalty.

Chicago police will once again be on hand in force to prevent violence in demonstrations outside the courthouse. In anticipation of the sentencing, both the Right to Youth movement and the God's Law Society were at the courthouse today. Several scuffles broke out. Eleven protesters were injured and were treated at the University of Chicago Megaplex Hospital before being released.

In related news, the board members of the Chicago Christian Health Network (CCHN) were meeting in Oak Brook. Reportedly on the agenda is the question whether CCHN should forbid its personnel to offer, refer for, or even recommend the Fountain of Youth therapy. Church authorities have urged such action, but CCHN executives have been sensitive to the economic implications of such a move. No report is expected from the board until next week at the earliest.

Study Questions

1. What might be advantages of a very long life for relationships? What might the disadvantages be?

2. Is the murder case an argument for marriage contracts of a limited term? In other words, is it imprudent for people with extremely long lives to commit to monogamous relationships?

3. It is imaginable that even if life-extending technologies become available that certain groups would decline to use them. If some groups use them and others do not, what ethical problems might emerge in terms of access to social goods such as political power, wealth, and so on? Would any of these problems be of a magnitude that would justify avoiding all research into life extension?

Prepared by Mark Waymack, Loyola University, Chicago, IL. Presented at the University of Illinois Science, Technology, and Society conference, "The Rejuvenator: Technology and the Transformation of Senescence," October 2000.

Rationing Health Care for Centenarians

With more people living longer and with medicine having more treatments to offer, the extent of health care for the elderly is facing serious debate. If everyone could be expected to live to at least 100 years of age, how would this affect existing arrangements in which the government provides health care for people above a certain age? One way to control costs would be to ration according to age. In the hypothetical example below, the proposal is to limit life-saving care to those under 100 years of age.

The *Chicago Sun-Times-Tribune*, *Oct. 20, 2057*: The U.S. Senate Committee on Health held a hearing Thursday to consider legislation that would deny Medicare reimbursement for life-saving health care interventions to anyone age 100 or older.

Due to widespread use of antiglucose, introduced to consumers some four decades ago, the United States now has 70 million centenarian. Although the agent enables body tissue to remain youthful and substantially expands life span and functional independence in old age, it does not make those who take it immune to life-threatening acute illnesses. As a result of the astounding increase in longevity, expenditures in Medicare have climbed from 2.5 percent of gross domestic product at the beginning of the century, to 20.3 percent today.

In his opening statement, committee Chairman Boris Frugal (R, Idaho) declared that continuing present Medicare reimbursement policies would devastate the economy. The lead witness, Dr. Justine Arbuckle, Murphy Professor of Biomedical Ethics at the University of Illinois at Chicago, declared, "It is essential and just to ration health care for centenarians."

Arbuckle praised the foresight of noted twentieth-century bioethicist Daniel Callahan. In his classic book published seventy years ago, called *Setting Limits: Medical Goals in an Aging Society*, he urged that life-saving care be denied to anyone eighty years of age and older because persons of this age have lived out their "natural life spans." Even before the advent of antiglucose, Callahan depicted the elderly population as a "new social threat" and a "demographic, economic, and medical avalanche . . . one that could ultimately . . . do great harm."

Arbuckle suggested that Callahan had set the age limit too low. "But using the age of 100," she said, "is certainly reasonable and necessary if our society is to survive. Now that we have the thirty-fourth amendment to the Constitution, weighting votes by age, it is also politically feasible to ration health care by age."

Thalma Witherspoon, president of the 60-million-member American Association of Centenarians, presented an opposing view. "Health care is a basic human right," she said. She asserted that it is essential to preserve the sanctity of human life at any age, "from the womb to the tomb."

Study Questions

1. The prospect of much longer life underscores the importance of government responsibility for health care. If it had no new sources of revenue, government resources could be considerably strained if people lived longer and increased the total amount of health care government was obliged to provide. Do you believe it would be ethical for a society, through the democratic process, to identify an age beyond which no life-saving health care would be provided? What age would that be?

2. Not all life-saving interventions cost the same. Some patients may require a short course of inexpensive antibiotics to ward off pneumonia. Others may require months of expensive care in intensive care units. Do you think it would be fair to use "life-saving intervention" as a benchmark for paying for health care?

Prepared by Robert H. Binstock, Case Western Reserve University, Cleveland, OH. Presented at the University of Illinois Science, Technology, and Society conference, "The Rejuvenator: Technology and the Transformation of Senescence," October 2000.

Offshore Rejuvenation

Together with research into the prevention and treatment of disease, researchers are working to identify the mechanisms of senescence. Control of these mechanisms could possibly extend either the productive years of a current human life span or the total number of years of life. The hypothetical case below raises issues that might develop should such advances be made.

The *Chicago Tribune, Oct. 20, 2022:* President Linda Scanlon met today with President Edmund Torres of the Cayman Islands, in an atmosphere of worsening relations. Evidence continues to surface that implicates the Cayman Islands in providing unregistered genetic rejuvenator therapy to Americans.

Any American who receives genetic rejuvenator therapy is required by law (OBRA 2019) to register such treatment with the US Department of Health and the Department of the Treasury. The "undocumented rejuvenated" are able to enjoy traditional Social Security and Medicare benefits, while at the same time living decades longer than their unrejuvenated peers.

As the American medical profession has become increasingly compliant in its reporting, there has been a steady increase of offshore rejuvenations, with the Caymans reputed to provide nearly 40 percent of them. The Cayman Islands, economically buffeted in recent years by significant loss of land to rising sea levels and a consequent decrease in tourism, has been eager to find alternative sources of revenue. Unregistered rejuvenating centers have sprung up, and policing has been lax.

President Scanlon says she is "very serious" about quashing such unregistered rejuvenations, but has said little about how she hopes to reduce—much less eliminate—them. Republicans, whose interest in supporting Social Security and Medicare waned some years ago when means testing was implemented, suggested either a gene-policing force to track down the unregistered rejuvenated or else getting the government out of Social Security and Medicare altogether.

Study Questions

1. What are predictable burdens on government if people live considerably longer?

2. Extension in longevity does not by itself mean an increase in health per se. People could live longer in a way that makes them susceptible to sickness as well. What effect do you think this might have on the way in which health care is paid for through insurance provided by employers or delivered by the government?

3. If genetic rejuvenation was possible, what ethical problems might spring up with regard to its availability and use? Would these problems be so serious that the techniques should not be used at all?

Prepared by Mark Waymack, Loyola University Chicago, IL. Presented at the University of Illinois Science, Technology, and Society conference, "The Rejuvenator: Technology and the Transformation of Senescence," October 2000.

5.16

Reading Your Mind

It can be instructive, as well as entertaining, to imagine what the future might be like if we develop certain technologies. What if a technology could read people's minds at a distance? Would this worsen antagonism between nations or force an openness that would reduce conflicts? Imagine, if you will, a world in which you could read others' thoughts at will . . . and they could just as easily read yours.

Neuroscientists are trying to relate specific brain functions to specific states of consciousness. We know that certain regions of the brain are associated with certain kinds of mental activities. When brains are damaged in a particular area, specific capacities can be lost. Is it possible to move beyond this general association to a more precise account? Could it be possible to identify specific brain functions that produce specific thoughts? For all the spies who might be interested in this science, could it be possible to use imaging techniques to read these thoughts? And, best of all, could this reading be done at a distance, for example, from a car parked outside the embassy of a hostile country? In 1998, the chairman of the French National Bioethics Commission raised a concern about the development of such technology. Jean-Pierre Changeux, who is a neuroscientist at the Pasteur Institute in Paris, said that such technology might become commonplace and could open the doors to massive invasions of privacy, posing "a serious risk to society."

Study Questions

1. To what extent do you believe it is important to conduct research into the association of particular brain functions with particular thoughts? What might the applications of such a science be?

2. What might the consequences be for the legal system if an individual's thoughts could be detected through examination of neurological function?

3. How desirable would it be to live in a society in which an individual's thoughts could be read directly and not merely just measured against his or her behavior?

Adapted from Jonathan D. Moreno, *Undue Risk: Secret State Experiments on Humans* (New York: W.H. Freeman, 2000), p. 293.

US Recruitment of Nazi Researchers

The collapse of Nazi Germany brought about the end of a horrendous chapter in human history. Some Nazi researchers were hanged for their crimes against humanity; others managed to make themselves attractive to nations bidding for scientific talent. The case below is representative of the kind of judgments made in the name of advancing US science.

For sixteen years, through the end of World War II, Hubert Strughold was director of Germany's Air Ministry's Aeromedicine Institute. He had finished a PhD and a medical degree, and was a pioneer in the study of the medical effects of air travel. During the war, both his superiors and subordinates were involved in studying the effect of immersing human beings in cold water for long periods. Some of these studies were carried out with prisoners from the infamous concentration camp Dachau. By every account, it is impossible for Strughold not to have known of these studies.

Yet the man was never charged, never arrested, and never prosecuted for war crimes. In fact, immediately after the war, the American director of the Heidelberg Institute put him to work collecting his colleagues' reports. In this capacity, Strughold wrote a study called "German Aviation Medicine: World War II." In 1946, a US Air Force colonel put Strughold's name on a list of German researchers to be brought to the United States. Strughold entered this country in 1947 and went to work at Randolph Air Force Base.

In response to a complaint in the mid-1970s, the US Immigration and Naturalization Service (INS) reopened Strughold's case for investigation with regard to possible war crimes. The agency closed the inquiry when a Texas congressman stated that the issue had already been thoroughly investigated. The INS admitted later that it had no evidence Strughold had ever been asked about his involvement in the low-temperature experiments.

In the mid-1980s, the Justice Department began efforts to prosecute Strughold as a war criminal, despite his being by now a much-honored aeromedicine expert in this country. Strughold was by this time medically infirm, which slowed interest in his prosecution. He died in 1986, never having been charged for inhuman experiments with prisoners.

Study Questions

1. What actions in biomedical research would justify excluding someone from entering the United States and becoming a citizen? On the evidence presented here, does Dr. Strughold meet those criteria?

2. Is knowledge that someone such as Dr. Strughold could bring to a research program so important that it might justify looking away from criminal wartime acts? It was sug-

gested that Nazi data should be used; might a similar case be made regarding Nazi scientific talent?

3. Do you believe that rehabilitation is possible that would make it acceptable for accused Nazi criminals to enter the United States and, after that, participate in its research programs?

Adapted from Jonathan D. Moreno, *Undue Risk: Secret State Experiments on Humans* (New York: W.H. Freeman, 2000), pp. 88–92.

When the Subject Is Afraid of the Researcher

One of the core principles of research ethics is that subjects may withdraw from a study for their own reasons. However, not all subjects are able to withdraw easily. The hypothetical case below involves a child, who cannot be said to have the same range of opportunities for withdrawal that an adult would have.

Professor Pamela Thompson is widely regarded as the expert in second-language acquisition by school children and preschoolers. She is nearing the completion of a study of preschoolers whose first language is Creole. The study involves identifying the way in which verbal interaction with classmates influences language acquisition.

Professor Thompson asks a graduate student, Allan Mathers, to observe the last child involved in the study. Mathers studied three such students during the previous semester and he looked forward to this experience. However, the little girl does not warm up to Mathers; in fact, two weeks into the study the four-year-old appears to be afraid of him. Mathers wonders if this is because he has one blue eye and one brown eye. Other children have noticed this, but none has been afraid of him. In any case, he is not sure this is the reason.

Things don't improve in the next week but they don't become worse either. Mathers wonders whether he should contact the girl's parents to learn whether she has said anything about him at home. The child's teacher warns him against doing so, saying that she has met the father and has the impression that he might confront the girl in a hostile way. The father wants his daughter to succeed and doesn't seem prepared to tolerate difficulties in school.

The teacher then tells Mathers that she does not think he should continue the study, since the child has resisted all his attempts at friendship. The teacher is worried that the child will become afraid of school if Mathers keeps trying to have conversations she does not want to have. The teacher hints that she will ask Thompson to take him out of the classroom.

Mathers wonders whether he should withdraw and report to Thompson that the child could not be brought around to cooperate. He knows that Thompson will be disappointed and maybe a little angry that he could not finish this study in a timely fashion. He wonders whether this failure might influence future jobs and recommendations. He honestly believes he could win the child's confidence if only given a little more time.

Study Questions

1. What responsibilities does Mathers have toward the child? Is her apparent fear of him, irrational as it might appear, a good reason for him to withdraw from the study?

2. Do you think it would be appropriate for Mathers to contact the parents and use information from them to help him establish a more trusting relationship with the child?

3. Student researchers frequently worry that substandard performance will hurt their evaluations and careers. How should Mathers balance his wish to avoid a harsh evaluation from his research supervisor with the reluctance of the classroom teacher and the child to have him continue the interaction?

Modified from a case prepared by Kenneth D. Pimple, PhD, Poynter Center for the Study of Ethics and American Institutions, Indiana University, Bloomington.

Abative Research

Most medical research focuses on identifying the cause of a particular problem. One approach shifts the focus away from the cause to methods of reducing the problem. This is referred to as abative, *meaning to lessen the effect. The perspective below offers a profound challenge to the way in which research money is allocated today.*

Among the many ways to approach a scientific problem, one is to ask what causes a particular ailment; however, finding the cause of the disorder is often extremely difficult, since it may have more than one cause. Nevertheless, most science proceeds as if we can approach isolated causes and do something about them.

Another way is to ask what reduces a particular problem. This strategy has not been sufficiently pursued by science. One feature of this approach is that it avoids certain ethical problems altogether.

For example, one way to learn whether large amounts of refined sugar cause health problems would be to ask people to consume more sugar and monitor them to see what happens. It is hardly ethical to ask people to assume unknown degrees of risk if they can be avoided. In this case, they could be altogether avoided by asking people to eat less sugar and monitoring whether those individuals had fewer health problems. This knowledge then could be applied to prevent a great deal of health problems. As another example, from the perspective of reducing ill health, it is of little value to study whether alcohol "causes" driving accidents. However, it does add much practical value to know whether required breathalyzer tests reduce accidents.

Abative research can be tested without the ethical problems of asking people to expose themselves to risk. It can be carried out in simpler terms, since we do not have to know exactly how the interventions work. Genetic research would remain viable, but it need not have great practical relevance. And prevention measures could be studied and compared with one another in quantifiable ways. In the long run, it is better to test preventive theories about what causes an abatement in problems than to try and localize single causes of complex health problems.

Study Questions

1. What is the main thrust of this analysis that research priorities are often fundamentally misdirected? How convincing is it?

2. What are other examples of research that might be focused on preventing and reducing diseases rather than on identifying causes and treatments?

3. To what extent do you think a focus on abative research would be incompatible with, or antagonistic toward, research dealing with causes and treatments?

Adapted from J. H. Renwick, "Analysis of Cause—Long Cut to Prevention?" in Dan E. Beauchamp, Bonnie Steinbock, eds., *New Ethics for the Public's Health* (New York: Oxford University Press, 1999), pp. 110–114.

5.20

Drugs for the Diseases of the Poor

Like other industries, pharmaceutical manufacturers look for profits from their investments. Some believe, however, that the industry should be mindful of social considerations when identifying research projects. In some instances, drug development may focus on diseases in countries with the most money to pay for treatments. This focus can overlook diseases and disorders across the rest of the globe.

At a meeting attended by approximately 15,000 people, Carl Feldman, president of the Biotechnology Industry Organization (BIO), said in summer of 2002 that the industry as a whole should develop a foreign policy if it was to avoid ethical and social controversies. The field had already received strong criticism for focusing on genetically modified crops, gene patents, and stem cells, and in many ways, a perception exists that it is not responding strongly enough to public concerns. He noted that tabloids have helped shape an unflattering perception of biotechnology.

Feldman encouraged researchers to publicize the way in which gene modification could help make crops more resistant to disease, something important to developing countries. He also urged the industry to develop medicines that would be useful in developing countries. For example, these might include oral or nasal vaccines that do not require refrigeration. He also called on government to introduce financial incentives that would spur research and development in that area.

To secure a better relationship with developing countries, Feldman also called for closer cooperation with the World Health Organization, international governments, and nongovernmental organizations.

Study Questions

1. Who is most likely to benefit from innovations in biomedicine and bioagriculture at the present time? In what way is this distribution of benefits morally problematic?

2. One way to spur interest in medications useful in developing countries is to give researchers additional years of patent protection. Do you think this is an appropriate step, or do you think this approach could work against broad availability of a medication?

3. Some developing countries have chosen to "break patents," which means they ignore legal restrictions on producing and making drugs available. These countries usually do so in the face of a pressing health need. Under what circumstances do you think it is appropriate for a country to ignore patents in the production of medication?

Adapted from Geoff Dyer, "Biotech Sector Urged to Focus on the Poor," *Financial Times,* 12 June 2002, p. 6.

6

Embryos, Fetuses, and Children

Introduction

Embryonic and fetal research holds great interest throughout our society. Descriptive research is useful to answer questions about how the fusion of gametes occurs, how embryos develop, how embryonic cells develop into particular organs and tissues, how developmental problems can lead to disorders, and so on. In the early twenty-first century, there is enormous interest in the study of human stem cells, cells that are either omnipotent or pluripotent, meaning that they can develop into all (omnipotent) or most kinds (pluripotent) of body cells. This research could lead to important advances in tissue therapy and organ replacement. Stem cells may be obtained either from very young human embryos (embryonic stem cells) or from certain tissues in adults. Fetal research, involving fetal cells and tissues usually obtained from voluntary abortions, is useful to researchers interested in physiology and vaccine development. Scientists are also interested in whether certain kinds of fetal tissue transplantation can help treat diseases such as diabetes in children and adults. Others are interested in fetal medicine, treatment of disorders while the fetus is still in utero.

Important differences inform moral theory regarding the status of embryos and fetuses, and these differences generate sharp controversy. Some attribute a moral status to human embryos and fetuses that would protect them from harmful research, that is, from research or treatment not intended to benefit them directly. According to this view, it would be morally acceptable to perform experimental surgery on a fetus in a woman's uterus if that intervention could be beneficial to the fetus. It would not be morally acceptable to conduct experiments on human fetuses or embryos in the laboratory to study tissue physiology and development. A related viewpoint involves the position that no human embryos or fetuses should be specifically produced for research purposes.

Other perspectives do not attribute moral status to embryos or fetuses that would protect them from being used in research. According to this view, embryos and fetuses lack the characteristics that entitle them to protection as human *persons*.[1] People in favor of this interpretation believe that research on embryos and fetuses is permissible even if it is not directed toward goals that will benefit the embryos and fetuses themselves. Some analysts believe that certain limitations, such as restricting research to early stages of embryo development, are justified, but for the most part they accept the use of embryos and fetuses in research.

Between these poles of interpretation are middle positions of all kinds, from acceptance of certain types of research with embryos and fetuses to rejection of others. Given the variety of positions, it is not surprising that it is difficult to reach an abiding consensus of national laws and policies in this area.

Research Politics

Heated political, moral, and religious debate has never been far from research involving human embryos and fetuses. Some key developments in the United States are worth mentioning to suggest the way in which political decisions have been made in this area.

In 1974 Congress adopted the National Research Act, which imposed a moratorium on federally funded fetal research. In 1975 the Department of Health, Education, and Welfare issued regulations that required researchers to treat all fetuses in utero in a way that minimized harm, regardless of whether or not women intended to carry their pregnancies to term. These regulations also required that research involving in vitro fertilization (production of embryos in the laboratory) be approved by an ethical advisory board. That board was allowed to expire in 1980, without having approved any applications. In effect, the government declined to support this research. These same laws and policies did not, of course, apply to researchers using private money, and studies proceeded in the private sector.

In 1991 President Clinton issued an executive order to allow federal funding for some research with fetal tissue, provided certain regulations were followed in obtaining those tissues. In 1994 the National Institutes of Health Embryo Research Panel proposed the use of human embryos for up to fourteen days after fertilization. The panel chose this time limit for two reasons: fourteen days seems to be the upper limit past which no twinning occurs. For some people this threshold suggests that embryo has an identity all its own. At fourteen days of development the primitive or neural streak begins to develop. This is the identifiable beginning of the nervous system, and many people believe this to be a relevant threshold in recognizing moral individuality.[2]

In 1996 Congress enacted a legislative ban on the creation of human embryos using federal money as well as a ban on federally sponsored research that involves injury or destruction of human embryos. In 2000, the National Institutes of Health sought and received a legal opinion that this ban did not apply to materials *derived from* human embryos. It therefore planned to fund studies of human embryonic stem cells provided those cells were derived without federal support. This policy was put on hold by a new presidential administration taking office. In the summer of 2001, President George W. Bush announced a kind of compromise: he would allow federal support of research involving some human embryonic stem cells; however, these cells had to be taken from cell lines that existed before his decision. Scientists would not be able to use cells taken from embryos after that date. Thus they would have no incentive to create new human embryos for stem cell research, at least as far as federal sponsorship is concerned.

Given the way that federal law and policies are susceptible to changes in political will, it is unlikely that the policies described here will be the last word on the topic. It should be remembered that even if the federal government does not sponsor research with human embryos and materials taken from embryos, such studies are permissible in many jurisdictions in the United States and around the world. In many jurisdictions, researchers are not bound by specific regulations about how to obtain, treat, and dispose of embryos and fetuses. Critics insist that the government should fund a broad range of research precisely to bring those efforts under federal regulations and guidelines.

Cloned Human Beings

Until recently, the cloning of human beings was discussed mostly in the realm of science fiction and faked history.[3] In 1997, Scottish researchers cloned a sheep by transferring the nucleus of a cell taken from an adult sheep.[4] The nucleus was implanted into a sheep ovum that had been stripped of its own nucleus; the implanted cell was then treated in a particular way, and it began to behave like an embryo. These embryos were implanted into a sheep's uterus, and eventually, after many, many failures, a lamb was born and grew to adulthood. Other animals have been successfully produced through this technique as well: mice, cows, goats, and so on. This process is known as somatic cell nuclear transfer (SCNT). Strictly speaking, these cloned animals are not exact copies of the adults: they differ with respect to a small amount of genetic material in the donor cell and the experiences they undergo during development. Nonetheless, they are sufficiently alike to speak of them as clones.

Biomedical applications of SCNT are of considerable scientific interest and importance. The technique could be used to produce virtually identical human embryos for research, which would be useful to many studies. These embryos could also be the source of stem cells, with particular genetic traits selected in advanced by researchers. If stem cells could be coaxed into developing into tissues and organs, researchers could prepare genetically identical (or nearly identical) tissues and organs for transplant. This could virtually resolve the weighty problem of immune system rejection of transplanted organs and tissues.

For all the importance of SCNT across biomedicine, it is the prospect of cloned human children that has captured the social imagination. One group declared that it has in fact cloned human infants. Indeed, we may be only a few sincere efforts away from this end. The ethical question is whether it is safe and wise to do it. By now, many have voiced their opinions on the safety and wisdom of cloning human beings.[5] In 1997, President Clinton issued an executive order barring use of federal money for the purpose. In 1997, the National Bioethics Advisory Commission recommended adoption of federal statutes prohibiting cloning.[6] As of this writing, however, the US Congress has not acted on that recommendation or any other proposal to ban SCNT for either research or for producing a human being, although some states have adopted such prohibitions. Perhaps it is no surprise that interest in the procedure has found outlets elsewhere. In 1998 researchers in North Korea said that they produced a human embryo by SCNT, but they did not allow it to develop for any length of time.[7] There has been no independent confirmation of that report. In 2001, US researchers at Advanced Cell Technology used SCNT to induce early human embryonic development. This company says it has no interest in producing human beings; its interest is in the therapeutic products that could be developed from embryonic stem cells produced with the technique.[8]

The right to conduct research is generally grounded in First Amendment protection of free speech and the related pursuit of knowledge. By extension, a strong argument holds that researchers have the right to study SCNT. Funding of that research is a separate question. Researchers are not entitled to spend government money for projects of their own choosing. In this matter, the democratic process remains the mechanism for such decisions. Federal money aside, many firmly believe that private researchers should be able to conduct privately funded research with human embryos and fetal tissues as long as no social harm is done. In other words, the state should not unduly regulate or impede the right to conduct privately funded research unless it has important reasons for doing so. As in all matters related to human cloning, it is likely that this debate will continue to roil.

Selecting the Traits of Children

The extent to which people may use emerging assisted reproductive technologies to have children and to choose the traits of their children is hotly debated.[9] Courts have interpreted the US Constitution as protecting decisions about having and not having children as a fundamental right. In striking down a state law authorizing sterilization of certain criminals, the Supreme Court decision of Skinner *v.* Oklahoma (1942) described the right to procreate as "one of the basic civil rights of man." Another Supreme Court case, Eisenstadt *v.* Baird (1972), held, "If the right of privacy means anything, it is the right of the individual, married or single, to be free from unwarranted governmental intrusion into matters so fundamentally affecting a person as the decision whether to bear or beget a child." Federal courts once struck down an Illinois law that prohibited experimentation on a fetus unless the experimentation might be therapeutic for the fetus. The court found that this law violated a woman's right to privacy in reproductive choices, saying that "within the cluster of constitutionally protected choices that includes the right to have access to contraceptives, there must be included . . . the right to submit to a medical procedure that may bring about rather than prevent pregnancy."[10]

Even though the right to bear children is considered fundamental, it is most clearly established as a matter of law for married, opposite-sex couples. The rights of single people are less well established. To date, moreover, court cases focused mostly on conventional methods of having children. For this reason, the legal entitlement to assisted reproductive technologies, including SCNT, is not entirely clear. The fundamental question for courts is whether unconventional forms of assisted reproduction are different from established ways of having children, different in ways that would justify limiting access to them.

A related question is whether parents may use interventions not just to have children but to have children of a particular kind. Is it within their moral right to have a child that is a clone of a beloved relative? Is it within their right to have a child of a particular gender? Of a particular sexual orientation?[11] What is the social impact if wealthy people are able to choose children with desirable traits whereas poor parents have no such options?

In 2001, a clinical diagnostic center, GenoChoice, put this information on its Web page (www.genochoice.com): "Thank you for considering GenoChoice to plan the future well-being of you and your family. My name is Dr. Elizabeth Preatner, a prenatal geneticist and embryologist here at GenoChoice. Using our state-of-the-art technologies, you can quite possibly ensure that your child's life may be free of such diseases as cancer, Alzheimer's, and heart disease—as well as conditions like obesity, aggression, and dyslexia. Our probes and DNA amplifiers can identify these negative genes and eliminate them in your child . . . all at the pre-embryonic stage! And you can even specifically choose genes that may determine favorable characteristics in your child. With the special help of GenoChoice, you can truly offer your progeny 'the best of nature . . . before you nurture!'"

Given the choice, many parents would probably find it attractive to have children that are free of disease, obesity, learning disorders, aggression, and cancer. In fact, many research initiatives are under way to identify and control other traits of children. The ethical question now at stake is the extent to which it is legitimate to choose traits through techniques such as preimplantation diagnosis of embryos or SCNT. In large measure, the debate must be set against the background consideration that this is an area in which parents already have enormous influence. Parents profoundly influence their children with regard to language, intellect, religious beliefs, life goals, political views, recreation habits, speech patterns, ambitions, table manners, educational goals, and so on. The relevant ethical question is whether or not traits parents would be interested in selecting through prenatal or early childhood interventions are materially different from those over which they already have great influence.

Certainly, many things may be said in favor of reproductive interventions to avoid disease in children. But that is not the last word on the subject since some people object to these interventions regardless of their beneficial effect. It can also be a blurry line for parents trying to distinguish disorders from merely undesirable traits. In either case, they are trying to confer an advantage on their children.

Ethical Issues Revisited

Disagreement exists about the uses of embryos, fetuses, and selecting traits of children because these are interpretive matters. This disagreement exists because there is room for it. This is not to say that these matters are unimportant or solely matters of taste. It is to say that they are open to different interpretations because there are different ways to perceive, value, and experience them.

Some ethical questions belong to a particular age, and some must be revisited time and again. For example, in the era when hemodialysis was experimental and costly, medical institutions faced hard questions of who would receive the treatment. Now, because the federal government pays for its use, hemodialysis machinery is no longer in short supply, and no one in this country agonizes about who is going to die for lack of blood cleaning. By contrast, certain ethical questions are more durable, such as whether it is appropriate for physicians to assist the suicide of their patients. Involving as it does issues about the way in which to value life and medicine, the use of human embryos and fetuses in research is one of those touchstone issues that people of each generation must reexamine for themselves. No amount of machinery or money will make these questions go away.

Just as no set of scientifically established facts can establish how people should interpret the status of embryos, fetuses, and children, neither can a set of scientific facts establish what traits will be advantageous to children in the future. In the past, for example, it might have been advantageous for some children to be aggressive and boundary testing; in the future those same traits might put children at a serious social disadvantage. The trait of cooperation might be more useful than aggression in the future, although we have no way to be perfectly sure: parents' choices about what is best for their children might not hold up over time. The extent to which parents are entitled to select the traits of their children is another question that is brought into sharp focus thanks to assisted reproductive technologies, and it is one that is not likely to go away except through a profound change in culture.

References

1. Michael Tooley, *Abortion and Infanticide* (New York: Oxford University Press, 1983); Gregory E. Pence, *Classic Cases in Medical Ethics: Accounts of Cases that Have Shaped Medical Ethics,* 3rd ed. (Boston: McGraw-Hill, 2002).

2. George J. Annas, Arthur L. Caplan, Sherman Elias, "Stem Cell Politics, Ethics, and Medical Progress," *Nature Medicine* 1999 (5): 1339–1341.

3. For one such faked account, see David M. Rorvik, *In His Image: The Cloning of a Man* (Philadelphia: J.B. Lippincott, 1978).

4. Ian Wilmut, Keith Campbell, Colin Tudge, *The Second Creation: Dolly and the Age of Biological Cloning* (New York: Farrar Straus Giroux, 2001).

5. Here are a few: Paul Lauritzen, ed., *Cloning and the Future of Human Embryo Research* (New York: Oxford University Press, 2001); Glenn McGee, ed., *The Human Cloning Debate,* 3rd ed. (Berkeley, CA: Berkeley Hills Press, 2000); Gregory E. Pence, ed., *Flesh of my Flesh: The Ethics of Cloning Humans* (Totowa, NJ: Rowman & Littlefield, 1998); Martha C. Nussbaum, Cass R. Sunstein, eds., *Clones and Clones: Facts and Fantasies about Human Cloning* (New York: W.W. Norton, 1998); Leon R. Kass, James Q. Wilson, *The Ethics of Human Cloning* (Washington, DC: AEI Press, 1998); and Gregory Pence, *Who's Afraid of Human Cloning* (Totowa, NJ: Rowman & Littlefield, 1998).

6. National Bioethics Advisory Commission, *Cloning Human Beings* (Washington, DC: National Bioethics Advisory Commission, 1997).

7. See www.gsreport.com/articles/art000012.html.

8. See www.cnn.com/2001/TECH/science/11/25/human.embryo.clone/.

9. John Robertson, *Children of Choice: Freedom and the New Reproductive Technologies* (Princeton, NJ: Princeton University Press, 1994).

10. Conference Committee on Fetal Research and Applications, *Fetal Research and Applications* (Washington, DC: Institute of Medicine), 1994.

11. Timothy F. Murphy, *Gay Science: The Ethics of Sexual Orientation Research* (New York: Columbia University Press, 1998), pp. 103–135.

Antipregnancy Vaccine

Against the background of an exploding world population, there is a great deal of interest in finding birth control methods that are easy to use and effective. One area of research is in immunology, which could be used by men or women. An example is an antipregnancy vaccine that would turn a woman's immune system against early processes of pregnancy. Not all contraceptives are equal, however, in the view of women who worry that some of them create health risks and make them vulnerable to political and technological manipulation.

The goal of antipregnancy vaccines is to find a way to render women's bodies indifferent to gamete production, fertilization, or implantation. If this could be achieved, key stages in the reproductive cycle could be broken.

Judith Richter maintained that these vaccines hold out an "unprecedented potential for abuse." First of all, they would work by, in effect, treating ovulation and conception as immune disorders. The risk is that actual autoimmune disorders could result in which the body reacts against its own substances. Richter wondered too, how these vaccines, intended to work for approximately a year to a year and a half, could be kept from creating permanent immune reaction against ovulation and pregnancy. Finally, this method cannot be ended immediately if harmful side effects occur.

Richter noted that most research into immunological methods of birth control is directed toward women. Vaccines represent yet another reproductive burden to be borne by women. Beyond that, with an antipregnancy vaccine women lose the degree of control they have with other contraceptives. In addition, the vaccine could easily be given to women without their knowledge or consent: its administration could be easy to conceal. Given the history of abuse in research, she said, it is wishful thinking to believe that scientists would administer the vaccine only with informed consent.

For these reasons, some women and professional organizations have urged the abandonment of further research into these vaccines, with 430 groups from 40 countries calling for a halt. These groups find that the vaccines do not meet the needs of women, and women themselves should set the agenda in plotting the future of birth control research. Women do not wish to be mere subjects of research. They want democratic technology and medical ethics, and the control of pregnancy should be rejected as primarily a matter of population control. According to Richter, "the preoccupation with population has resulted in a conceptual framework in which birth control methods are seen not as an entitlement of people but as a weapon in the 'war on population' in which people are treated as mere numbers and statistics to be controlled, manipulated, reduced and dispensed with. In the process, women and men have become numbers and statistics and have lost their human faces." Antipregnancy vaccines not only heighten risks to women, they also feed into an objectionable ideology of birth control.

Study Questions

1. How important is it to develop antipregnancy vaccines? What would their advantages be? Their disadvantages?

2. Many people foresee misuse of an antipregnancy vaccine. Is this reason enough not to investigate the vaccines?

3. Do you think that interest in an antipregnancy vaccine is really a diversion from more important ways of addressing choices about having and not having children?

Adapted from Judith Richter, *Vaccination against Pregnancy: Miracle or Menace?* (London: Zed Books, 1996).

Pregnant Men

The topic of pregnant men bounces around the media from time to time. It is often presented as a joke or a far-fetched movie plot. In fact, some evidence suggests that men could gestate children. The possibility raises a variety of ethical questions.

In rare instances women have gestated children through placental attachment to the intestine. This occurred when the embryo somehow drifted into the abdomen and implanted there. Among such cases was the 1979 birth of a child in New Zealand to a woman who had no uterus at all. Other cases are documented in the biomedical literature. The placenta itself produces a number of hormones necessary for development, and cesarean section is performed to remove the child at the appropriate gestational age.

This biological occurrence led some researchers to believe that men could gestate children in a similar fashion. An embryo could be somehow attached to the intestine and given the additional hormones important to development. The infant would be removed through an abdominal incision, much as in cesarean section. Risks to the man would include bleeding from the implanted placenta and possible breast development from hormones.

Some fertility experts claim they have been approached for this service. In one instance, a woman lost her uterus, but not her ovaries, in an accident. The couple wanted to have in vitro fertilization to produce an embryo, but did not want to employ a surrogate mother. The husband was willing to try to gestate the child. It is speculated that male couples might also have an interest in gestating children.

The chairman of a British fertility association said of male gestation that "it is not ghoulish in any way, and you certainly could not stop a man from doing this in legal terms on the grounds of sex because that would be discrimination." Others reject the idea. A physician who helped pioneer in vitro fertilization, Ian Craft, said of male gestation that "it would be dangerous and is a distortion of nature." Another individual pointed out that the world had many more important issues to be worried about with regard to the existing state of fatherhood without adding gestation to the list.

Study Questions

1. Is anything inherently unethical about a man gestating a baby? Is there a reason it should never be done by any man anywhere?

2. The first child gestated this way would attract worldwide attention. Is this necessarily harmful to the child?

3. What is human nature, and why do some critics think it forms the basis for objecting to male gestation of a baby?

Adapted from Steve Farrar, Karen Bayne, *Sunday Times* [London], Feb. 21, 1999. See also John Money, *Gay, Straight, and In-Between: The Sexology of Erotic Orientation* (New York: Oxford University Press, 1988).

6.3

Political Compromise on Stem Cell Research

During the Clinton administration, the National Institutes of Health implemented a policy that would allow federal funding for some research on stem cells derived from human embryos. Before studies were conducted, this policy was suspended in 2001 by the incoming administration of George W. Bush. In summer of 2001 President Bush announced that funding could be used for this research provided that the stem cells in question were already available in cultivated cell lines. Research on cells from other embryos would not be permitted. An excerpt from the address Mr. Bush made to announce his decision is given below.

"My administration must decide whether to allow federal funds, your tax dollars, to be used for scientific research on stem cells derived from human embryos. A large number of these embryos already exist. They are the product of a process called in vitro fertilization, which helps so many couples conceive children. When doctors match sperm and egg to create life outside the womb, they usually produce more embryos than are planted in the mother. Once a couple successfully has children, or if they are unsuccessful, the additional embryos remain frozen in laboratories.

"Some will not survive during long storage; others are destroyed. A number have been donated to science and [are] used to create privately funded stem cell lines. And a few have been implanted in an adoptive mother and born, and are today healthy children.

"Based on preliminary work that has been privately funded, scientists believe further research using stem cells offers great promise that could help improve the lives of those who suffer from many terrible diseases—from juvenile diabetes to Alzheimer's, from Parkinson's to spinal cord injuries. And while scientists admit they are not yet certain, they believe stem cells derived from embryos have unique potential. . . .

"Embryonic stem cell research is at the leading edge of a series of moral hazards. The initial stem cell researcher was at first reluctant to begin his research, fearing it might be used for human cloning. Scientists have already cloned a sheep. Researchers are telling us the next step could be to clone human beings to create individual designer stem cells, essentially to grow another you, to be available in case you need another heart or lung or liver.

"I strongly oppose human cloning, as do most Americans. We recoil at the idea of growing human beings for spare body parts, or creating life for our convenience. And while we must devote enormous energy to conquering disease, it is equally important that we pay attention to the moral concerns raised by the new frontier of human embryo stem cell research. Even the most noble ends do not justify any means.

"My position on these issues is shaped by deeply held beliefs. I'm a strong supporter of science and technology, and believe they have the potential for incredible good—

to improve lives, to save life, to conquer disease. Research offers hope that millions of our loved ones may be cured of a disease and rid of their suffering. I have friends whose children suffer from juvenile diabetes. Nancy Reagan has written me about President Reagan's struggle with Alzheimer's. My own family has confronted the tragedy of childhood leukemia. And, like all Americans, I have great hope for cures.

"I also believe human life is a sacred gift from our Creator. I worry about a culture that devalues life, and believe as your president I have an important obligation to foster and encourage respect for life in America and throughout the world. And while we're all hopeful about the potential of this research, no one can be certain that the science will live up to the hope it has generated.

"Eight years ago, scientists believed fetal tissue research offered great hope for cures and treatments—yet, the progress to date has not lived up to its initial expectations. Embryonic stem cell research offers both great promise and great peril. So I have decided we must proceed with great care.

"As a result of private research, more than 60 genetically diverse stem cell lines already exist. They were created from embryos that have already been destroyed, and they have the ability to regenerate themselves indefinitely, creating ongoing opportunities for research. I have concluded that we should allow federal funds to be used for research on these existing stem cell lines, where the life and death decision has already been made.

"Leading scientists tell me research on these 60 lines has great promise that could lead to breakthrough therapies and cures. This allows us to explore the promise and potential of stem cell research without crossing a fundamental moral line, by providing taxpayer funding that would sanction or encourage further destruction of human embryos that have at least the potential for life.

"I also believe that great scientific progress can be made through aggressive federal funding of research on umbilical cord placenta, adult and animal stem cells which do not involve the same moral dilemma. This year, your government will spend $250 million on this important research.

"I will also name a president's council to monitor stem cell research, to recommend appropriate guidelines and regulations, and to consider all of the medical and ethical ramifications of biomedical innovation. This council will consist of leading scientists, doctors, ethicists, lawyers, theologians and others, and will be chaired by Dr. Leon Kass, a leading biomedical ethicist from the University of Chicago. This council will keep us apprised of new developments and give our nation a forum to continue to discuss and evaluate these important issues. As we go forward, I hope we will always be guided by both intellect and heart, by both our capabilities and our conscience."

Study Questions

1. Do you think this policy reflects a consistent moral approach to the use of human embryonic stem cells? Does it demonstrate uniform treatment of human embryos, or does it have

more in common with political compromises and show evidence of trying to reconcile incompatible moral views?

2. Researchers believe that many human stem cell lines now available will not be useful. They believe that some of them do not reproduce in a reliable way or that they will be of little value in treating particular diseases. They also believe that they will be eclipsed in importance by new stem cell lines being developed in the private sector. It is indeed likely that many new cell lines not in existence at the time of President Bush's decision will become available. Do you think that the logic of Bush's decision could justify expanding the pool of stem cell lines that federal researchers could be permitted to use?

3. This policy does allow researchers to conduct both federally sponsored and privately sponsored research in the same laboratories. It allows researchers to use embryonic stem cell lines created after the president's decision, as long as that research is paid for with nongovernment money and as long as the funds are not commingled. Does this policy violate or abide by the spirit of the president's decision to restrict federally sponsored research to existing cell lines?

Quoted from www.whitehouse.gov/news/releases/2001/08/20010809-2.html. See also Clive Cookson, "Most Stem Cell Lines 'Will Prove to be Unviable,'" *Financial Times*, June 12, 2002, p. 6; and Sheryl Gay Stolberg, "U.S. Rule on Stem Cell Studies Lets Researchers Use New Lines," *New York Times*, Aug. 7, p. 1.

No Embryonic Stem Cell Research

In 2000 the National Institutes of Health drew up guidelines for funding some human embryonic stem cell research. Various groups protested because this would involve destruction of human embryos. They also claimed that the research was scientifically unnecessary given that researchers have other methods for obtaining stem cells for medical purposes. The following statement captures some of the ethical objections to embryonic stem cell research.

"The prospect of government-sponsored experiments to manipulate and destroy human embryos should make us all lie awake at night. That some individuals would be destroyed in the name of medical science constitutes a threat to us all. Recent statements claiming that human embryonic stem cell research is too promising to be slowed or prohibited underscore the sort of utopianism and hubris that could blind us to the truth of what we are doing and the harm we could cause to ourselves and others. Human embryos are not mere biological tissues or clusters of cells; they are the tiniest of human beings. Thus, we have a moral responsibility not to deliberately harm them . . .

"The last century and a half has been marred by numerous atrocities against vulnerable human beings in the name of progress and medical benefit. In the nineteenth century, vulnerable human beings were bought and sold in the town square as slaves and bred as though they were animals. In this century, the vulnerable were executed mercilessly and subjected to demeaning experimentation at Dachau and Auschwitz. At mid-century, the vulnerable were subjects of our own government's radiation experiments without their knowledge or consent. Likewise, vulnerable African Americans in Tuskegee, Alabama were victimized as subjects of a government-sponsored research project to study the effects of syphilis. Currently, we are witness to the gross abuse of mental patients used as subjects in purely experimental research.

"These experiments were and are driven by a crass utilitarian ethos which results in the creation of a sub-class of human beings, allowing the rights of the few to be sacrificed for the sake of potential benefit to the many. These unspeakably cruel and inherently wrong acts against human beings have resulted in the enactment of laws and policies which require the protection of human rights and liberties, including the right to be protected from the tyranny of the quest for scientific progress.

"The painful lessons of the past should have taught us that human beings must not be conscripted for research without their permission—no matter what the alleged justification—especially when that research means the forfeiture of their health or lives. Even if an individual's death is believed to be otherwise imminent, we still do not have a license to engage in lethal experimentation—just as we may not experiment on death row prisoners or harvest their organs without their consent. . . . Of all human beings, embryos are the most defenseless against abuse. . . . The intentional destruction of some human beings for the alleged good of other human beings is wrong."

Study Questions

1. Is the analysis persuasive that there is no important reason to use human embryos as the source of stem cells?

2. Do you accept the view that we all have the duty not to harm any human embryos intentionally?

3. Is the analysis persuasive that human embryos should not be conscripted into research without their consent? Is it meaningful to talk about embryos giving consent?

Downloaded from "Do No Harm" Web page (stemcellresearch.org) July 30, 2000. This excerpt is taken from "On Human Embryos and Stem Cell Research: An Appeal for Legally and Ethically Responsible Science and Public Policy." The text was accompanied by a request to reprint the document only in its entirety (which is not done here) and to acknowledge the Center for Bioethics and Human Dignity as author (which I am happy to do).

Research on Human Embryos

Considerable debate surrounds the topic of using human embryos for research. As is well known, it concerns not only the moral status of embryos but also use of taxpayer money for the research. Critics believe that those who oppose this experimentation should not be required to pay for it with their taxes.

Critics fault the government for failing to fund human embryo research in meaningful ways. They point to the value of such research for overcoming infertility, for producing useful tissues, and for developing treatments for debilitating conditions. Gregory E. Pence, a bioethicist at the University of Alabama at Birmingham, said, "Many clinics have hundreds, even thousands of human embryos stored in liquid nitrogen. If these embryos could be used for research that prevented even one kid from having cystic fibrosis or Tay-Sachs disease, wouldn't it be worth it?

"A fourteen-day-old embryo the size of the period at the end of this sentence is a far cry from an eight-month-old human fetus. Why is it morally valuable to protect hundreds of such non-feeling human embryos? Why, if the cost of this protection is one, or twenty children born with Down's syndrome, cystic fibrosis, or degenerative neurological diseases? Isn't such embryo worship idolatry? Because embryos don't perceive anything or feel pain, isn't their value purely rhetorical and symbolic?"

Pence also noted that a ban on federally supported study of human embryos for therapeutic purposes has fueled research in the private sector. He says that every year perhaps one million couples pay for some assistance at fertility clinics. The desire for children fuels a huge industry of privately controlled and largely unregulated research on human embryos. Unwanted embryos may be donated for research by private companies in many national and international jurisdictions.

Study Questions

1. What reasons might there be for research involving fetal tissue? How important do you think this line of research is?

2. Do you think that government money should be made available for research on human fetuses and embryos, research about which there is divided moral opinion?

3. What do you think of the view that human embryos have only a rhetorical and symbolic value and that they may therefore be used to help protect people from debilitating and degenerative diseases?

Adapted from Gregory E. Pence, *Re-Creating Medicine* (Lanham, MD: Rowman & Littlefield, 2000), pp. 71–74.

Access to Reproductive Cloning

The cloning of many kinds of mammals—sheep, mice, cows—provoked consider-able public resistance to the idea of performing SCNT to produce a human being. After that initial response came more modulated responses that opened the door— at least a bit—to the idea. One philosopher concluded that reproductive cloning is ethically defensible, but only for infertile couples who cannot produce a genetically related child in another way.

Carson Strong, professor of medical ethics at the University of Tennessee, is not convinced by some of the standard objections raised against cloning. He does not believe that it poses an undue threat to the uniqueness of individuals. A cloned child will have its own experiences and life. He thinks, too, that cloning might be per-formed safely, if not immediately then eventually. Neither does he believe that it is necessarily a threat to the parent-child relationship or that it would lead to objectifi-cation of children. He is also skeptical that totalitarian regimes would be able to use the technique to great advantage.

Because he thinks safety difficulties can be managed, he makes a case that cloning should be made available to infertile couples who want a child genetically related to at least one of the parents. He says specifically that it is morally defensible for use by couples who have tried and failed all other methods of having a child.

Cloning is justified, he says, because it extends the couple's desire to participate in the creation of a person and affirms the mutual love between the man and woman. It also opens up the possibility of the experience of pregnancy, childbirth, and child rearing. For all these reasons, Professor Strong believes that if it can be done safely, SCNT should be available to these specific infertile couples. In the analysis as he first presented it, he made no reference to same-sex couples or single parents.

Study Questions

1. What is the main argument here about why SCNT may be used in some instances to have a child?

2. Do you believe this professor has a convincing reason why SCNT may be performed only for couples who have tried and failed to have children by other assisted reproductive technologies?

3. Do you think that other persons—not mentioned here but including perhaps same-sex couples and single women and men—are also entitled to use SCNT to have a child? Why or why not?

Adapted from Carson Strong, "Cloning and Infertility," *Cambridge Quarterly of Healthcare Ethics* 1998 (7): 279–293. See also Timothy F. Murphy, "Entitlement to Cloning," *Cambridge Quarterly of Healthcare Ethics* 1999 (8): 364–368.

Obtaining Fetal Tissue for Research

The following commentary points out that abortion can be linked to the way in which human fetal tissue is obtained. This linkage is worth considering for its own ethical implications about appropriate ways in which to obtain research materials.

Human fetal tissue has been used in privately funded research for several decades. Researchers hope that transplantation of this tissue will help improve the function of impaired thymus and parathyroid glands, liver, pancreas, and brain. The success of such transplantations is still uncertain, but is being studied.

Abortion is a mainstay for acquisition of tissue for this purpose, and using anencephalics (babies born without brains) is explored from time to time as well. One ethical question is whether the need for tissue influences the way that abortions are performed. The state of the tissue is very important for transplantation, and for this reason certain abortion techniques are preferred over others.

For example, hysterotomy involves the surgical removal of the fetus through an incision in the abdomen. In contrast, prostaglandins may be used to induce labor and achieve termination of pregnancy. From the point of view of the tissue researcher, the former technique is preferable because tissue is less damaged. Another technique of abortion, suction evacuation of the uterus, is even less desirable, because it can be difficult to pick out the target tissue. Instead, it is possible to put a woman under general anesthesia, introduce a suction tube into the uterus under ultrasound guidance, and remove target fragments of the fetal body without contaminating them with other tissues.

It seems, therefore, that the interests of fetal tissue research can influence the way that abortions are conducted, not only how they are carried out, but also the gestational age of the fetuses. Indeed, the very possibility of fetal tissue research can be an inducement to abortion insofar as the public is concerned: if people believe that this tissue can be put to good use, that is one more reason to accept abortions.

Study Questions

1. Is anything inherently unethical in selecting one abortion technique over another to retrieve tissue in a particular condition?

2. It is suggested that abortion may be influenced by researchers' desire for tissue in a particular state. What kind of conflict of interest might this introduce into the clinical experience of women having abortions? Do you believe that women who schedule abortions are entitled to know if any aspect of their experience is influenced by research needs?

3. Do you agree that the public will be more accepting of abortion if it understands that fetal tissues are put to good use in research?

Adapted from Peter McCullagh, "Some Ethical Aspects of Current Fetal Usage in Transplantation," in Peter Byrne, ed., *Ethics and Law in Health Care Research* (Chichester: John Wiley & Sons, 1990), pp. 25–43.

6.8

Fetal Death and Tissue for Research

The use of fetal tissue is morally controversial in itself, and the means to obtain this tissue adds another layer of complexity to the debate. The discussion below raises questions about inconsistencies in the way the death of human beings is determined and how fetal tissue is obtained.

The incentive to formulate a uniform determination of brain death was driven by interest in obtaining organs for transplantation. As a matter of law and ethics in the United States, a person is considered dead if the body lacks key neurological functions. The body can lack these functions and still be apparently alive in that respiration and blood circulation continue through mechanical assistance. This standard applies across all people regardless of age, identity, and social status.

Yet in the case of fetuses, it might not be possible to achieve consistency in making determinations of death. For example, fetuses may be aborted by hysterotomy, which involves their removal by an incision in the woman's abdomen and uterus. This can produce a fetus capable of living for a time outside the uterus. Brain death cannot be measured in these bodies in the same way it is measured in other human bodies. What standard of death, therefore, should be applied in such instances, especially if researchers are interested in using tissue from fetuses?

The standard definition of brain death requires that body temperature be greater than 35°C. If the body is not at least this warm, the low temperature may reduce the heart rate so that it is undetectable. A fetus outside the uterus cannot maintain body heat so it takes on the temperature of the environment. But maintaining its body temperature at 35°C or higher could threaten the usefulness of the tissues taken after confirmed death. In contrast, if the fetus is cooled to protect the value of the tissues, the diagnosis of cardiac cessation would not reveal whether cardiac death properly speaking has occurred. Therefore, a question of consistency is raised in determining death. Inconsistency that reduces public confidence in the fairness and objectivity of standards of death may undermine support for fetal tissue research.

Study Questions

1. In the United States and elsewhere, brain death is accepted as both the legal and ethical standard of death for human beings. Bodies in this condition require no medical treatment, and organs and tissues may be taken from them. Do you find it worrisome that determination of fetal death may not be consistent with standards in adults and children?

2. Worries exist about excising tissue and organs from fetuses that are not definitively known to meet standards of brain death. To what extent are they a good reason to forbid using tissues and organs from this source?

Adapted from Peter McCullagh, "Some Ethical Aspects of Current Fetal Usage in Transplantation," in Peter Byrne, ed., *Ethics and Law in Health Care Research* (Chichester: John Wiley & Sons, 1990), pp. 25–43.

Freezing and Transplanting Ovary Tissue

Studies of the physiology of reproduction make it possible for people with gamete problems to have genetically related children. Researchers are looking at more effective ways of preserving human eggs. One way to do this is to implant ovarian tissue into women. Although no child has yet been born this way, researchers are optimistic that successful efforts with animals will carry over to humans.

By themselves, female gametes (eggs) do not freeze well, making it difficult to store them for later use. Some children have been born from frozen eggs, but the success rate is very low. However, it appears that strips of ovarian tissue that contain hundreds or thousands of immature eggs can withstand freezing.

Scientists are investigating this technique as a way of maintaining a woman's eggs for a substantial period of time. Roger G. Godsen of McGill University took strips of ovarian tissue from mice and sheep, froze them, thawed them, and reimplanted them. The eggs that ripened within the animals were extracted and used successfully to produce healthy offspring. The freezing and implantation technique also produced healthy eggs in monkeys, and might work with humans.

A researcher at Cornell University Medical School, Kutluk Oktay, removed ovarian tissue from two women (although the tissue was not frozen) and transplanted it back into their bodies under the skin of their forearms, rather than in the pelvic area. This location was chosen because it did not require extensive surgery or general anesthesia, and was easy to monitor for disturbances and disorders. The implanted tissue produced not only mature eggs but monthly hormone effects.

It is thus possible that women could freeze a portion of their ovaries and reintroduce it into their bodies later as a way of delaying or eliminating menopause. The technique might also be effective in women who face chemotherapy or radiation that could damage their ovaries. The tissue would be removed before therapy and reimplanted after it was finished. Physicians might also remove ovarian tissues for freezing if a woman wanted to delay childbearing.

Dr. Oktay tried to fertilize three human eggs retrieved from tissue implanted in the arm of one woman, but the attempt was not successful. It is unclear how long the hormonal effects of implanted tissue might last. It is also unclear how many women might wish to pursue such an intervention.

Study Questions

1. What are some reasons women might wish to have samples of their ovarian tissue excised, stored, frozen, and possibly reimplanted in their bodies later on?

2. Does this line of research open up new reproductive possibilities in a way that potentially harms the status of women? For example, would this technology, like others, possibly rein-

force the idea of women as valuable only insofar as they have children? In what other ways might this technique work against the interests of women?

3. What information would be essential to the informed consent process if researchers should begin clinical trials to learn whether formerly frozen reimplanted ovarian tissue can produce eggs capable of resulting in a child?

Adapted from Lila Guterman, "An Armful of Eggs: Ovarian Transplants Could Restore Lost Fertility," *Chronicle of Higher Education*, Jan. 26, 2001, p. A19.

Placebos in Research with Children

Federal regulations governing research with children call for due consideration of risks and potential benefits. Researchers may conduct studies that involve no greater than minimal risk to children, that involve greater than minimal risk if the risk is justified by possible benefit to the children, and that involve a minor increase over minimal risk but are justified not in terms of direct benefit to individual subjects but in terms of important knowledge about children's disorder or condition. Under certain conditions federally sponsored or regulated researchers may conduct studies that do not meet these conditions, but only after review by a specific panel and approval from the Secretary of Health and Human Services. In the case below, researchers propose an experimental treatment for newborns in a study that involves a placebo intervention.

"Based on a series of pilot studies, investigators suspect that prolonged administration of a new monoclonal antibody will prevent episodes of systemic *Staphylococcus* infection in premature infants. The investigators propose a randomized, double-blind, placebo-controlled trial in which premature infants will be given daily intramuscular injections of the study drug or placebo. Principal outcome measurements of the study include evidence of infection by blood culture and number of days of hospitalization following birth per infant."

Walter Robinson maintained that this study of infants does not need a placebo control. Some animals seem to show a placebo effect, but the prevailing view is that the effect requires some cognitive powers such as assigning meaning and causation to sickness, understanding the nature of research and treatment, discriminating between treatments, and forming expectations of interventions. Because they have no such capacities, premature infants are unlikely to exhibit the placebo effect.

Robinson proposed that the study only has to blind the researchers. "For the purposes of this trial, a small bandage at the (presumed) injection site should have the same observer-blinding effect as an actual injection of saline: the observer could not tell which infant is getting what treatment. Such a maneuver would accomplish the goal of blinding the observer without inflicting pain on the infant." Even if a placebo effect did exist, he maintains that the main outcomes of the study—blood culture findings and days of hospitalization—are not especially sensitive to the placebo effect.

Study Questions

1. Federal regulations governing research with children call for due consideration of risks and potential benefits. Do daily injections of a placebo impose unacceptable risks for the babies?

2. Is the statement that babies do not exhibit the placebo effect convincing? What further information or evidence might be necessary to determine the truth of this position?

3. How might the effect of the monoclonal antibody be tested in another way to determine its value?

Adapted from Walter M. Robinson, "Ethical Issues in Pediatric Research," *Journal of Clinical Ethics* 2000 (11): 145–150.

Designer Children?

More than ever, children's traits are under the control of parents. Some parents already face choices about genetic and developmental disabilities in their children. It is expected that more and more choices will become available with regard to all children. This expectation of choice has led to questions about the extent to which parents might want to "design" their children.

Prenatal examinations can ascertain whether an embryo or fetus will be male or female. Amniocentesis and ultrasound can identify a variety of genetic and developmental disorders. Other screening tests, such as blood tests, can identify problematic development. All these methods can allow parents to avoid having children of a certain kind. For in vitro fertilization, an unwanted embryo is not implanted into a woman's uterus. If fetuses are detected with unwanted traits, they can be aborted. There is every reason to think that biomedicine will offer more control over the traits of children, especially as more discoveries are made about the foundations of traits such as intelligence, height, curiosity, and so on.

Some commentators see the increasing power of prenatal intervention as a threat to the sanctity of human life. People worry that parents will carry out a kind of eugenics against children with traits they consider undesirable. They worry that parents will shift from wanting healthy children to superior children. In addition, social pressure may force parents, women especially, to avoid having a child with an unwanted trait. The desirability of traits is culturally determined, and what is desirable in one culture may not be desirable in another, but the availability of technology may foster misconceptions about what is best for all children.

In contrast, it is noted that parental influence over children is already profound in the realms of language, religion, culture, habits, dispositions, politics, and so on. Thus control over other traits is merely an extension of acceptable moral practice. According to this view, if parents want to choose a trait that will confer some advantage on a child, why shouldn't they be able to? If parents can choose to give their children an expensive education to help them get ahead, why shouldn't they also be able to choose how tall their children will be?

Study Questions

1. Is it ethical for parents to select the gender of their children through such techniques as in vitro fertilization, embryo transfer, or selective reduction during pregnancy?

2. Would it be ethical for parents to use prenatal techniques to select an embryo or fetus believed to have superior intelligence?

3. In what way, if any, is employing biomedical interventions to shape children's traits different from teaching them multiple languages, sending them to superior schools, and cultivating certain political views in them?

6.12

What Counts as Disease?

Some children are short because of identifiable disorders that interfere with normal growth. Other children are just short; they have no obvious disorders and are perfectly healthy. However, shortness has cultural disadvantages, and many parents do not wish their children to be short. Increased knowledge about the role of growth hormones has led to treatments for children whose height is stunted by pathological disorders. However, those same treatments appear attractive to parents of children who are short but healthy.

Some disorders that interfere with production of growth hormone cause short stature in humans. They can often be treated with exogenous growth hormone, that is, hormone from a source outside the individual. For short stature that is not related to these disorders, however, there is no recommended medical treatment. Growth hormone can still be administered to such children, but that practice is a matter of debate.

Critics claim that administering exogenous growth hormone to short but healthy children is not ethical because short stature is not a disease. It is not ethical to submit children to treatment risks even if they (and their parents) enthusiastically agree to it. Short individuals are not functionally diseased, but they may be at risk for psychological difficulties. Nevertheless, it is difficult to know whether height will increase a particular individual's success and happiness.

Much medical research is not for diseases properly speaking, such as studies of aesthetic surgery. Proponents of growth hormone treatment claim that happiness and success in this society are linked to height, so successful treatment would provide benefits beyond mere height increase. They do concede, however, that risks of medical management are a real concern in conditions that are not diseases. On balance, they recommend that children who are short, even if not for a medically identifiable reason, be treated with growth hormone.

Study Questions

1. In what sense is height important for a meaningful human life? Are you convinced that an important difference exists between short stature that is caused by a disease and short stature that is simply part of the human range of height?

2. Is short stature so problematic that it justifies exposing healthy children to the risks of hormone treatment?

3. In a parallel treatment, physicians administered estrogens to suppress the growth of tall girls. In high dosages, estrogens arrest elongation of the bones, but reports associate this treatment with reproductive complications. Do you believe this is an appropriate use of estrogens with these risks or even without risks?

Adapted from Ruth Macklin, "Growth Hormones for Short Normal Children: An Ethical Analysis," *American Society for Bioethics and Humanities Exchange* 1999 (2): 1. Further information and debate may be found at the Web site of Physicians Committee for Responsible Medicine; see www.pcrm.org, "Research Controversies and Issues."

Deaf Culture and Babies

A great deal of ethics analysis has focused on applying reproductive technologies to confer an advantage on children. A central question is whether this will turn children into commodities and deepen the divide between rich and poor. However, it is not always clear how advantage is to be defined. In the case below, a couple succeeded in having a child who is significantly deaf. The case provokes questions about the nature of disabilities and the extent to which parents may select traits in their children that interfere with a major life function.

Sharon Duschesneau and Candace McCullough have been in a relationship for ten years, and have one daughter, age five. They agreed to let a reporter from the *Washington Post* interview them and be present at the birth of their next child. Ms. Duschesneau has severe hearing loss, and Ms. McCullough is profoundly deaf. What makes their story interesting is that in trying to have children, both women agreed to increase their chances of having a deaf child. They see their deafness as an identity, not as a deficit. When they approached a sperm bank with this interest, they were told that deaf men are excluded as donors. The women therefore turned to a deaf friend with a family history of extended deafness, for sperm for insemination. Their first child is deaf, and their next child has only residual hearing in one ear. Neither of the women sees their actions as bringing a child with a disability into the world. They see their children as being another kind of normal. They are aware, too, that their children will be eligible for social service benefits, and believe it will be less costly for them to have deaf children than to have hearing children.

Both women are concerned about the social fate of deaf people in a time when screening and other reproductive techniques can work in the favor of parents who do not want deaf children. Ms. McCullough responds to the worry that there will be no more deaf children in the future by noting that other people such as she and her partner will choose to have such children.

Study Questions

1. Do you believe it is defensible for parents to try to increase the odds of having a deaf child?

2. What are the disadvantages of deafness, and are they so severe that parents should never try to have a deaf child?

3. The Americans with Disability Act defines a disability as an impairment of a major life function. That interpretation extends to deafness. Do you believe it would be appropriate to interpret parental decisions to achieve a disability in their child as abuse?

Adapted from Liza Mundy, "A World of Their Own: In the Eyes of His Parents, if Gauvin Hughes Turns out to Be Deaf, That Will Be Just Perfect," *Washington Post*, March 31, 2002, p. W22.

6.14

SmartKid

Whether or not genetic interventions should be used to improve children is one of the enduring ethical questions in genetic research. As the case below shows, this question can arise even if the interventions are only preliminary and carried out in nonhumans. Implications for human beings are extremely important as they relate to a key trait and value.

In 1999, Princeton University scientist Joe Z. Tsien added a gene to a mouse named Doogie. This gene enhanced the brain's NMDA receptors and improved the mouse's learning and memory significantly. The increased intelligence stayed with the mouse as it grew.

Dr. Vivienne Nathanson, head of the ethics section of the British Medical Association, warned that this experiment "leads to the specter of designer babies and the concept of children being rejected because they do not have these qualities."

Steven Rose, head of the brain and behavior group at Great Britain's Open University, stated, "This is a real piece of vulgar hype from Princeton. They shouldn't do this stuff; it really is irresponsible . . . Human intelligence is something that develops as a part of the interaction between children and the social and natural world, as they grow up. It is not something locked inside a little molecule in the head."

In contrast, bioethicist Gregory Pence of the University of Alabama at Birmingham observed that people should probably not assume that the first and most important use of such a discovery would be the improvement of normal human children. The discovery could hold important benefits for autistic children or those with developmental disorders. It might even be effective for treating Alzheimer disease or other such conditions. Where's the harm, he asked, in helping parents find treatments for conditions that keep children out of school and even institutionalized?

Study Questions

1. How important is this line of research? What might some of its applications for animals (or humans) be?

2. Is this research really irresponsible? Do you think that researchers should not conduct experiments with animals (or humans) to study ways in which to enhance intelligence?

3. If this research showed promise for humans, is there any reason why it should not be studied with regard to enhancing intelligence in normal people as well as those with some degree of mental impairment?

Gregory E. Pence, *Re-Creating Medicine* (Lanham, MD: Rowman & Littlefield, 2000) pp. 105–107.

7

Genetic Research

Introduction

Many biomedical researchers believe that the study of molecular biology will transform medicine and bring untold benefits to the public health.[1] For example, some commentators have described AIDS as a genetic disease.[2] They do not doubt that it is caused by HIV infection, but note that certain people are immune for genetic reasons. If researchers can reproduce this immunity in others through a genetic intervention, they will have found a protection against the disease. Another example concerns protection not from disease but from senescence, with manipulated genomes perhaps leading to longer and more vital lives.[3]

Whereas genetic research defines many landmarks in biomedical progress, it is still an armchair game for speculating about what the future will be like when research consolidates its achievements into effective applications. At the present time, we stand at the threshold of an unforeseeably vast horizon of biological knowledge. The roots of contemporary genetic medicine may be in preventing and controlling disease, but it takes only a short leap of imagination to recognize that these efforts offer control of other traits as well, intelligence, physical size, and appearance among them, and not only for humans.

Progress in Genetic Research

Much early genetic research was focused on the origins of specific diseases such as cystic fibrosis, hemophilia, and Huntington disease. Although keen interest remains in locating genes associated with those diseases, the multinational Human Genome Project (HGP) has now described the human genome.[4] The word "genome" refers to the full genetic complement of an organism, and the HGP produced a functionally complete genome of human beings and several other organisms (some bacteria, yeast, fruit flies, etc.). These organisms were chosen to help develop the technology for mapping and sequencing and because they held promise in uncovering the way in which genes function. With available technologies, the genome of any organism can be fully described. Whether researchers will wish to do this will depend on the value of compiling these vast libraries of information.[5]

Even though we have a functionally complete map of the human genome, it is not well established what each element does or how its parts interact with each other. Therefore, the medical benefits of the HGP are still modest. In the main, applications of genetic research will be experimental for some time to come. Virtually no genetic treatments for human disease are available in the sense that physicians can modify the genome of an individual to relieve a disease or disorder. Various effective treatments (nutrition, drugs, etc.) relieve symptoms but do not alter their underlying cause. In the immediate present, the primary significance of genetic research for medicine is likely to be an increase in information about specific individuals. The power to test for genetic traits has opened a variety of ethical questions. So pressing are questions about privacy, confidentiality, and the meaning of genetic traits, that a portion of the HGP was devoted to consideration of its ethical, legal, and social implications.[6] Many of these issues are explored in the cases in this chapter.[7]

Experimental Genetic Medicine

A key focal point of genetic research is to identify means of altering genes in organisms, including people. In the mid-1960s discoveries showed that the DNA of viruses insinuated themselves into the DNA of human cells and changed the functions of those cells. This discovery is the basis for thinking that intentional changes can be made to human DNA. The mechanism for introducing new DNA into human DNA is called a vector. Possible vectors for introducing altered DNA include treating cells outside the body and reintroducing them into the body, injecting treated cells into a particular organ, and injecting altered cells or viruses into the body in the hope that they will migrate to the appropriate area.

The primary ethical concerns in this venture are those associated with any frontier medicine. Because so many aspects of this research are unknown, informed consent and proper selection of subjects become difficult. Research in identifying a vector to treat a particular condition was responsible in 1999 for the death of an eighteen-year-old man who had been treating his genetic disorder successfully through diet and drugs. Together with others, he participated in a study to learn whether a particular vector could be used safely in human beings. Because the study was about the vector, not about its effect, it was not expected that he would benefit. In fact, he became seriously ill and died quickly. Some contended that consent was inadequate in this study. It was also questioned whether researchers would have done better to choose gravely ill babies who had little hope of recovery from their disease rather than adults whose illness could be controlled through treatment.[8]

Are risks of genetic interventions different from risks people face in other biomedical research? In fact, other research can carry grave risks to health, and it is hard to make the case that genetic research is entirely different. Nevertheless, what sets this work apart is that it tries to alter functions at the lowest level of causality in an organism. These interventions may become routine and safe one day in the future, but given the present state of knowledge, it is reasonable to proceed with caution and in ways that minimize the damage of experiments should they go wrong.

Germ-Line Interventions

One key distinction that guides much discussion in genetic ethics is the difference between somatic and germ-line interventions. The distinction can be described in the following way. Suppose a genetic intervention is developed that allows the liver of a human being to produce an enzyme it could not produce before, for example, by introducing altered cells into the liver that would produce the missing enzyme. This would be a treatment confined only to the particular individual. Because the change would not be replicated in this person's gametes, his or her children would still be at risk of inheriting the enzyme deficiency. Thus, somatic interventions affect the individual but are not heritable. In contrast, germ-line interventions are heritable and can be passed along to future generations. Many agree that somatic interventions are acceptable but that germ-line interventions should not be carried out because of their unknown effects.[9]

Despite this concern, an important germ-line boundary was crossed in 2001. Clinicians at two fertility clinics announced that they had produced children using human eggs to which a small amount of DNA from another woman had been added as a way to overcome infertility. The eggs were then fertilized with sperm. This is a good example of a germ-line intervention insofar as the children produced this way show genetic lineage from three parents, and that lineage will be passed to their children.[10] It was undertaken without review by an independent ethics body and without public discussion. It remains to be seen whether it will result in damaging consequences in the long run.

Social Effects of Genetic Medicine

One of the primary effects of genetic research will be to increase the information available about an individual. Some tests will identify not only the root cause of existing disorders but also identify *predictors* of disorders that may occur later on in life. In theory, a child could be tested at birth—or even as an embryo or fetus—

for known genetic diseases that manifest themselves throughout life. To be sure, many of these predictive tests are inconclusive in the sense that they estimate only a general likelihood that a disorder will or will not emerge. Nonetheless, a good deal of damage could be done if children were tested and they or those around them saw only disorder and disease ahead in their lifetime.

It is not only affected individuals who would be interested in knowing their future health. Genetic predictors of disorder and disease are of keen interest to employers and insurers as well. Because of the potential for discrimination, the consensus is that genetic testing should be conducted primarily to identify exactly what disorders a person may have or may reasonably be expected to have. In other words, it should be considered a clinical tool rather than as an indicator of eligibility for insurance, employment, or military service. Needless to say, many challenges lie ahead to ensure that these procedures primarily benefit the individual rather than social institutions.

Over and above risks to particular individuals, some are concerned that genetic interventions will affect social groups, for example, those defined by race, ethnicity, geographical isolation, or other factors that may predisposed people to genetic disease and result in stigmatization.[11] Another concern is that genetic research will deepen the social divide between haves and have-nots. Once treatments are widely available, people who can afford them will be better protected, and thus they and their children will have advantages most other people would lack.

Some commentators point out that genetic interventions will help comparatively few individuals, and it might be better to put the money used for this research elsewhere. For example, social resources could be diverted to public health purposes such as cleaning toxic environments, providing preventive medical care, or even keeping water supplies clean. These efforts would improve the health of considerably more people than genetic medicine could.

Genetics and Children

An expected benefit is that genetic research will extend reproductive choices available to parents. Thousands of diseases are caused by alteration of a single gene, and potential parents, gametes, embryos, and fetuses can be tested for many of these genes. This expands parents' choices considerably. If they are shown to be carriers of a genetic disease, they can avoid having children altogether. In conjunction with in vitro fertilization and embryo transfer, gamete selection or embryo testing can be performed to conceive children who do not have genetic disease. Of course, it is not possible or always prudent to test for all genetic diseases. New mutations will also thwart efforts at detection. It is perhaps too obvious to state that many people will not have access to genetic technologies during the conception and birth of their children. For these reasons, children will continue to have genetic diseases.

Not all parents make the same choices when facing the possibility of genetic disease in their children. For example, some hold that assisted reproductive technologies such as in vitro fertilization and techniques of pregnancy termination are immoral, and they often stress the need for finding treatments rather than enhancing mechanisms for preventing the birth of affected children. Chapter 6 contains a number of entries dealing with the effects of genetic research for preventing disease in children and in choosing other traits. The question of selecting traits that confer an advantage on children, as against avoiding disease in children, are some of the most contentious questions about genetic interventions.

Beyond Human Beings

Many implications of genetic research extend beyond human beings. Engineering of animals and plants is a major concern in research ethics. Early research with bacteria and viruses raised considerable fears that transgenic organisms might be harmful to human beings. One fear was that early recombinant DNA techniques might produce harmful pathogens that could escape from the laboratory and kill people. This concern was addressed in the seminal 1975 Asilomar conference, at which participants called for a moratorium on recombinant DNA research until such time as safety precautions could be put in place.

In fact, a good deal of biomedical research depends on transgenic organisms, plants and animals alike. Moreover, the United States and other countries permit the patenting of transgenic plants and animals.[12] Bacteria, plants, and strains of lower-order animals are all protected under patents as long as they are shown to be nonhuman, multicellular, alive, and not naturally occurring. The predominant view is that it is ethically acceptable to produce these organisms as long as it is done safely and as long as potential dangers to the environment are controlled. This is easier said than done. Transgenic organisms could well disrupt established balances in nature, giving some plants or animals a survival advantage. Moreover, if humans exert strong genetic influence over plants and animals, the gene pool of these organisms might narrow, putting them at risk. For example, if most wheat were produced using one transgenic stock and that stock later proved susceptible to a killer virus, the world might be at risk of extremely serious food shortages. That risks of this kind exist does not mean that it is necessarily wrong to produce transgenic organisms. What it means is that their production and use should be monitored closely to identify and prevent such problems.

Using transgenic organisms to produce food for humans is an issue that is far from settled.[13] Some critics call genetically modified food "Franken-food." In fact, many foods already on the market come from genetically modified sources. This debate first caught fire in Europe, but its concerns are applicable everywhere, namely, that too many genetically altered foods have been introduced without public notice and appropriate testing. One concern, among others, is that reliance on genetically modified crops and foods will enlarge the powers of multinational corporations to control what humans eat. Others contend that genetically modified food will help resolve world hunger.[14]

References

1. Nicholas Wade, *Life Script: How the Human Genome Discoveries Will Transform Medicine and Enhance Your Health* (New York: Simon & Schuster, 2001).

2. LeRoy Walters, Julie Gage Palmer, *The Ethics of Human Gene Therapy* (New York: Oxford University Press, 1996).

3. McGee, Glenn, ed., *The New Immortality: Science and Speculation about Extended Life* (Berkeley, CA: Berkeley Hills Books, 2002).

4. Cook-Deegan, Robert, *The Gene Wars: Science, Politics, and the Human Genome Project* (New York: W.W. Norton, 1994).

5. Murphy, Timothy F. "Ethical Aspects of the Human Genome Project," in Helga Kuhse, Peter Singer, eds., *Companion to Bioethics* (Oxford: Blackwell, 1998), pp. 198–205.

6. See Daniel J. Kevles, Leroy Hood, eds., *The Code of Codes: Scientific and Social Issues in the Human Genome Project* (Cambridge: Harvard University Press, 1993); Timothy F. Murphy, Marc A. Lappé, eds., *Justice and the Human Genome Project* (Berkeley: University of California Press, 1994); and Phillip R. Sloan, *Controlling our Destinies: Historical, Philosophical, Ethical, and Theological Perspectives on the Human Genome Project* (South Bend, IN: University of Notre Dame Press, 2000).

7. See also Allen Buchanan, Dan W. Brock, Norman Daniels, Daniel Wikler, *From Chance to Choice: Genetics and Justice* (New York: Cambridge University Press, 2002).

8. Julian Savelescu, "Harm, Ethics Committees, and the Gene Therapy Death," *Journal of Medical Ethics* 2001 (27): 148–150.

9. LeRoy Walters, Julie Gage Palmer, *The Ethics of Human Gene Therapy* (New York: Oxford University Press, 1997).

10. Gina Kolata, "Babies Born in Experiments Have Genes from 3 People," *New York Times*, May 5, 2001.

11. See Raymond A. Zilinkas, Peter J. Balint, eds., *The Human Genome Project and Minority Communities* (New York: Praeger, 2002); and Barbara Katz Rothman, *The Book of Life: A Personal and Ethical Guide to Race, Normality, and the Implications of the Human Genome Project* (Boston: Beacon Press, 2001).

12. David Magnus, Arthur Caplan, Glenn McGee, *Who Owns Life?* (Buffalo, NY: Prometheus Press, 2003).

13. See Martin Teitel, Kimberly Wilson, *Genetically Engineered Food: Changing the Nature of Nature*, 2nd ed. (Rochester, VT: Inner Traditions International, 2001); and Gregory Pence, *Designer Food: Mutant Harvest or Breadbasket of the World?* (Totowa, NJ: Rowman & Littlefield, 2002).

14. For a discussion, see Per Pinstrup Andersen, Ebbe Shioler, *Seeds of Contention: World Hunger and the Global Controversy over Genetically Modified Crops* (Baltimore: Johns Hopkins University Press, 2001); and Robert L. Paarlberg, *The Politics of Precaution: Genetically Modified Crops in Developing Countries* (Baltimore: Johns Hopkins University Press, 2001).

7.1

Asilomar

Gene transfer provoked a great deal of discussion about the ethics of recombinant techniques and their social consequences. Perhaps some of this discussion was due to the rise of ecological consciousness in the United States in the early 1970s, and perhaps some was due to journalistic lapses and oversimplifications. Nonetheless, the ability to transfer genetic material from one organism to another had important implications for human safety. Public concern certainly played a role in a moratorium geneticists imposed on recombinant DNA techniques.

In the summer of 1971 researchers planned studies with SV40, a monkey virus that can induce cancerous growth in monkey and human cells. The news media drew attention to plans to introduce DNA from this virus into bacterial cells of *Escherichia coli*. These bacteria are present in the human intestinal tract, and if these experiments went wrong, it was possible that pathogenic bacteria could escape from the laboratory and kill humans who lived nearby. The techniques of DNA transfer opened up a staggering number of possibilities of gene combination. Because of public reaction to this new horizon of science, SV40 research was postponed. In fact, in 1973 and 1974, prominent scientists, including a committee of the National Academy of Sciences, called for a temporary halt to such studies until safety and procedural issues could be addressed.

In 1975 the National Institutes of Health sponsored a conference at the Asilomar Conference Center in California, entitled "International Congress on Recombinant DNA Molecules." Biologists, physicians, and attorneys met to discuss the safety of recombinant DNA research, focusing not on ethical issues of genetic alteration but on safety and public reassurance. Numerous questions were addressed: could dangerous pathogens escape into the environment? would recommended guidelines be enough to protect workers and the public, or were formal regulations required? The conference concluded that such research could go forward, but only after certain safeguards were implemented, including sterilization and containment mechanisms.

Study Questions

1. The conference at Asilomar was held at a time when recombinant DNA techniques were new, but no harmful transgenic organisms had been created and released into the environment. As no harm had been done, is it possible that the public and researchers panicked and imposed an unnecessary moratorium?

2. The moratorium on recombinant DNA study is virtually without precedent in scientific history. Are there other domains of research that might benefit from a moratorium until guidelines and/or regulations are developed to deal with potential problems? What factors would have to be present for a moratorium request to be successful?

Adapted from Marcia Baranaga, "Asilomar Revisited: Lessons for Today?" http://www. biotech-info.net/asilomar_revisited.html.

Germer-Line Therapy

The HGP produced a functionally complete map and sequencing of the human genome. The map identifies the constituent genes of human beings and several other organisms, and sequencing identifies the nucleotide base pairs that make up those genes. Even before these features were functionally complete, considerable speculation surrounded the future of genetic interventions. One debate that has been simmering since the early twentieth century concerns germ-line interventions. These would not only modify the genetic endowment of somatic cells, but would alter germ cells and be carried into future generations. This debate has become more pitched as the prospect of meaningful genetic interventions grows closer.

In somatic genetic interventions, only a given person's genetic function would be altered, not heritable traits in the person's gametes. For example, if a man's diabetes were controlled through a somatic genetic intervention, he would still be capable of passing along a genetic disposition to diabetes to his children.

Germ-line interventions would control the genetic trait not only in the individual, but also in his or her gametes. Some consider this objectionable in the extreme on the grounds that if something were to go wrong in the person, that same damage would be inflicted on future generations. For example, control of a genetic disposition toward diabetes might contribute to an increased susceptibility to cancer. Critics see no need whatsoever for this sort of intervention, because prenatal diagnostics and treatments could meet all the needs of germ-line therapy. In the case of diabetes, a physician could diagnose a genetic susceptibility to the disease at birth and begin to treat the child.

Another objection to germ-line therapy is that it would widen an already broad divide between rich and poor. If the therapy is expensive, and it would likely be, its benefits would not be available in an equitable way. In addition, it would likely be used to enhance people rather than merely to prevent disease. For example, if genes related to superior cognitive abilities are discovered, rich people might use germ-line interventions to ensure having bright children, which is not the same thing as protecting them from disease or disability.

Germ-line therapy could also aggravate the debate about research on human embryos. Study of the safety and efficacy of these interventions in humans would no doubt require considerable numbers of human embryos.

The prospect of controlling the fate of future human beings raises questions and fear. It seems better to leave the fate of people to chance rather than concentrate it in the hands of one person or group. In other words, there are boundaries to intervention that no human should cross. A more concentrated version of this view suggests that germ lines could be controlled for malevolent purposes, comparable with Nazi racial hygiene programs.

A final argument is that children have the right to receive a genome that has not been tampered with by anyone.

Study Questions

1. What are the chief worries about germ-line interventions?

2. How convincing are proposals that there should be no germ-line interventions?

3. How likely is it that germ-line therapy will contribute to a sharper division between haves and have-nots?

4. It is really true that children have the right to expect a genome that has not been planned by anyone?

Adapted from LeRoy Walters, Julie Gage Palmer, *The Ethics of Human Gene Therapy* (New York: Oxford University Press, 1997), pp. 60–98.

ELSI Projects

The HGP devoted part of its budget to the study of ethical, legal, and social implications (ELSI). This component is intended to identify and prevent various social problems. Consider the case below not only for the problem under analysis, but also as an opportunity to determine whether the analysis is able to help identify and prevent social problems.

The Environmental Genome Project parallels the HGP in many ways but focuses on interactions between genes and the environment. Richard R. Sharp and J. Carl Barrett maintain that the point of the Environmental Genome Project's ethical, legal, and social implications (ELSI) arm is to "anticipate potential problems before they arise and to develop policies that maximize the benefits of the research while avoiding potential misuses of the information learned." They believe that the project will raise problems that are not like those that genetics usually involves.

For example, they suggest that we are fairly well equipped to deal with ethical questions about rare, highly penetrant genetic conditions that occur only infrequently and are profoundly evident. Because those disorders are not easily treated, they are singled out in social policy on grounds that they are different, that they lead to objectionable treatment, and that people who have them are often unable to modify their situation. For these reasons, ethics strongly supports strict control over access to genetic information.

This viewpoint may not be as clear or as compelling for other kinds of genetic susceptibilities. Sharp and Barrett believe that the advance of environmental genome research will identify common genes of low penetrance. Therefore, strict control over genetic information may not be as important, since discrimination is less likely if large numbers of people have the same condition. If these people do face discrimination, it is much more likely that they can join together and effect a political solution to the disorder. Moreover, they may be able to avoid many problems simply by changing their environment, such as by removing a toxin or by moving away.

Therefore the potential benefits of collecting and disclosing genetic information may outweigh limited risks of discrimination. "Though commentators on genetic research involving highly penetrant alleles are correct in highlighting the potential for discriminatory uses of genetic information, it is not obvious that these considerations apply with the same force to polymorphisms in common genes of low penetrance."

Study Questions

1. How convincing is it to say that when it comes to widespread genetic dispositions to disease, confidentiality is less important for affected parties?

2. Do you think it is true that the democratic process will allow people sharing widespread genetic traits to disease to avoid objectionable social treatment in employment, housing, and so on?

Adapted from Richard R. Sharp, J. Carl Barrett, "The Environmental Genome Project and Bioethics," *Kennedy Institute of Ethics Journal* 1999 (9): 175–188.

Environmental Genome Research

The study of the relationship between the environment and individual genomes is expected to make significant strides in the years ahead. The Environmental Genome Project is a government-sponsored effort to describe ways in which genes and the environment interact. As it does, it will raise questions about how to respond to health problems associated with both genetics and the environment.

The Environmental Genome Project will attempt to "assemble a set of DNA samples that reflect the genetic diversity of the US population and to make a set of immortalized cell lines for the identification and study of genetic polymorphisms." Polymorphisms are variations within standard genetic profiles. Of particular interest are polymorphisms that "metabolize or detoxify chemicals," such as those that "alter an individual's ability to process a specific chemical, to respond to a given environmental exposure, or to repair DNA damage." In this regard, the project will examine environmental interactions with individual and multiple genes, as well as gene interactions with other genes.

One question that arises with regard to this project is what constitutes an adequate genetic sample of the United States population. Should this be carried out across gender lines, ethnic groups, and age groups? Should immigrants be included, as well as people born in the United States?

Of more substantial ethical concern, what standard of informed consent should prevail when taking new samples from people, or samples from existing immortalized cell lines? Because the specific uses of these samples is not yet predictable, how can consent be informed? And if people cannot be given this information, what exactly are they consenting to when they agree to give a sample?

The project also raises questions of notification regarding one's own polymorphisms. Should people who donate samples be told if research shows that they have polymorphisms that make them particularly susceptible to an environmental toxin? This question is even more problematic because many of these findings will be cast in probabilistic terms. That is, studies may show that 10 percent of people with a particular polymorphism develop disease in the presence of a particular environmental toxin, but most people do not.

Study Questions

1. What standards of consent should be involved in any effort of this kind? Do you think a blanket consent to any and all uses is fair, or should consent be limited to specific, identified uses if subjects remain identifiable through future studies?

2. What standard of notification should be involved in such an effort? Do you believe researchers have obligations to notify subjects if they find genetic dispositions to disease?

Adapted from Richard R. Sharp, J. Carl Barrett, "The Environmental Genome Project and Bioethics," *Kennedy Institute of Ethics Journal* 1999 (9): 175–188.

7.5

The Specter of Eugenics

Advances in genetic research have been viewed skeptically by some people who see the agenda being chosen without involvement of any meaningful democratic process. Others raise the concern that the research will engineer a master class of human beings. The following passage is taken from a larger text calling for people to join public interest groups as a way of making research initiatives answerable to the people.

"Just as biotechnology is changing the gene structures of plants, animals, microbes, etc., eugenics alters people. After the Human Genome Project completed sequencing the human genetic structure, the media loudly trumpeted the presumed medical benefits of re-engineering hereditary human characteristics. But most media left out the likelihood that human genetic alteration would be used for other purposes such as: 'More desirable cosmetic, emotional, or mental traits. (Tall, blonde, blue-eyed? Smarter? Dumber? Submissive? Can work long hours?) Ultimately, the use of eugenics may depend on fashion, or worse; who's in charge.' 'Designer babies' are possible. So are 'chimeras,' part human/part animal. Someday will someone seek to create and clone a superior new race? It's been proposed before. Princeton's Dr. Lee Silver, an advocate of human genetic engineering, predicts that society might eventually be divided into genetic classes: the 'naturals' who have not been genetically improved, and the 'GenRich' (about 10% of society). The GenRich will run businesses and institutions while the naturals are laborers. Since these genetic changes will become part of the hereditary germline, class divisions will be permanent. So, where do you stand on this? Has anyone ever asked?"

Study Questions

1. To what extent does this commentary fairly represent the issues at stake with regard to researchers' and public's involvement? Is it a fair assessment?

2. How convincing is the view that a class of the "GenRich" will run the world at the expense of the "naturals?"

3. What would "asking" the public about future uses of genetics involve? In other words, what kind of public involvement would make the uses of genetics less objectionable than they are represented here?

Source: "Techno-Utopianism" [advertisement], Turning Point Project, *New York Times*, Aug. 28, 2000, p. A11.

Secondhand Smoke

Genetic research will undoubtedly reveal traits that make some people more suscepti-ble to environmental toxins and effects than others. Certain individuals, for example, may be especially susceptible to skin cancer associated with sunlight. Others may be more susceptible to toxins in water or soil. These results will raise questions about the responsibilities of individuals and society. Who has the responsibility to protect individuals from environmental influences: those who have the genetic susceptibility or society at large?

The goal of the Environmental Genome Project is to identify genetic traits that mark-edly increase the risk of developing certain diseases in certain environments. Suppose that several genetic polymorphisms are identified that significantly increase the risks associated with secondhand smoke. People with these genetic variations are highly susceptible to lung cancer and emphysema that are usually associated with tobacco smoke. Their susceptibility has a genetic component, and is not merely a function of being exposed to environmental smoke.

What measures would be appropriate for identifying these people? Would it be fair to mandate that parents who smoke screen their children for these polymorphisms in order to keep smoke away from the children? Would they be guilty of neglect or abuse if they did not accept the genetic screen, or if they found these polymorphisms in their children but did not stop smoking themselves? Could divorce courts making custody determinations conclude that one parent would be a better parent because he or she did not smoke? Would it be fair to extend genetic testing to employment for work in taverns, bars, and other venues where smoking is permitted?

Perhaps most important, would it be fair for health insurers to deny coverage to smokers on the grounds that they knowingly accept the risk of smoking, that they could avoid disease later on but choose not to? Would failure to protect against geneti-cally predictable disease come to be seen as genetic irresponsibility, leaving it fair game to exclude such people from employment, insurance, and other social benefits?

Study Questions

1. If genetic disposition to cancer is associated with exposure to secondhand smoke, do par-ents who smoke have a duty to test their children for that disposition?

2. Do you think it is reasonable to introduce smoking into divorce proceedings, again on the assumption that one parent may smoke while the other does not, and assuming that children may be disposed to cancer from exposure to secondhand smoke?

3. Do you think that the increasing discovery of genetic dispositions to disease set the thresh-old of responsible parenthood ever higher, perhaps too high?

Adapted from Richard R. Sharp, J. Carl Barrett, "The Environmental Genome Project and Bioethics," *Kennedy Institute of Ethics Journal* 1999 (9): 175–188.

7.7

Patented Organisms

The advent of genetic manipulations of organisms inevitably raised the question of patents for such organisms. Patents secure the right to make, license, or sell the item in question, and some genetically modified organisms are of considerable commercial interest. Until recently the US Patent Office had no history of dealing with such organisms. When first approached on the matter, it rejected the attempt to patent a modified bacterium. The US Supreme Court set that decision aside, opening the door to the patenting of all manner of living organisms.

Patents are secured for new, useful, and nonobvious processes. In the 1980 case of Diamond *v.* Charkrabarty, the US Supreme Court held that genetically modified organisms could be patented as items of manufacture or new composition. The justices affirmed a broad interpretation of congressional intent in developing patent law. They asserted that Charkrabarty's bacterium did not exist in nature but was a creation of the inventor, and that it had a novel character and use. It was modified to help break down crude oil and would thus be useful in cleaning up oil spills.

In 1988 the US Patent Office granted a patent on a genetically engineered mouse that contained a gene that made it highly susceptible to cancer, and thus was useful in testing suspected cancer-causing substances. This precedent opened the door for patents on all kinds of organisms whose genes have been modified for one reason or another.

The Patent Office was not persuaded by various objections to these patents, in particular, the assertions that these genetic modifications violated the organism's natural integrity. Biologists do not claim that there is a specific boundary for the borders of a species. Moreover, species exhibit many genetic changes in nature; their genomes are not fixed forever. Finally, it is unclear species have moral right to remain unchanged forever. Nevertheless, the public still sometimes expresses concern about the nature and limits of genetic modification of organisms.

Study Questions

1. Do boundaries of nature in organisms exist such that humans should not produce transgenic animals that combine genes from more than one species?

2. The right of patent gives the researcher licensing control over the use and production of such organisms. Do you agree that it is wise to allow researchers to patent new organisms? Or should such organisms be in the public domain to be produced and used as the public wishes?

3. How convincing is the view that no organism—no animal, no plant—has the right to remain genetically unchanged forever?

Adapted from US Congressional Office of Technology Assessment, *New Developments in Biotechnology: Patenting Life* (Washington, DC: US Government Printing Office, 1988).

Therapy versus Enhancement

Some people believe that genetics should not be used to improve human beings in ways that do not involve the alleviation of disorders or diseases; for example, to produce taller or smarter children. The proper use of genetics is to free human beings from the burden of disease. However, as discussed below, protection from disorders may entail genetic interventions of a kind that make the distinction between alleviating disease and improving humans beside the point.

The literature on the ethics of genetic interventions tends to accept a distinction between therapy and enhancement. Therapeutic interventions are designed to remedy some disorder, such as diabetes or cancer. Enhancement interventions are designed to improve a trait, such as intelligence. Some scientists put emphasis on interventions and do not accept the legitimacy of enhancements. They see the work of genetics as curing disease, not improving humans.

However, environmental genetic efforts may undo this distinction and the moral priority given to therapeutic genetics. For example, environmental genetics may reveal that some people are particularly disposed to skin cancer by reason of a common genetic polymorphism that has low penetrance. Therefore people with this trait might want genetic intervention to avoid the effect of the polymorphism. They could choose to alter their environment and reduce the amount of sun to which they are exposed, but they would rather alter themselves.

Moreover, because of low penetrance of the polymorphism, not all of these people would be at significant risk of skin cancer, but they might not wish to take that chance. At the same time, they might wish to live in a sunny climate and go to the beach as often as they can. It is unclear that a genetic intervention with such people would be therapeutic per se, because they might never show symptoms and might never develop the illness in question.

Study Questions

1. How credible and useful is the distinction between therapeutic and enhancement uses of genetics?

2. If people are discovered to have genetic dispositions to disease, would it be fair for health insurance to draw distinctions among them according to those dispositions? For example, if people with a disposition toward skin cancer continue to live in sunny Florida rather than wintry Minnesota, might insurers not ask for more money for coverage of these Floridians?

3. Do you think that the emphasis on finding genetic dispositions to disease might influence policy makers to "punish" individuals through exclusionary practices? For example, might social policy identify and remove susceptible workers from toxic workplaces rather than clean up the workplaces?

Adapted from Richard R. Sharp, J. Carl Barrett, "The Environmental Genome Project and Bioethics," *Kennedy Institute of Ethics Journal* 1999 (9): 175–188.

Consent and Assumption of Risk in Genetic Therapy

What is the role of IRBs in evaluating the choice of subjects in research? One way to select subjects is to choose adults in preference to children on the theory that they are better situated to understand risks. It is preferable to avoid vulnerable subjects (especially those diminished with regard to capacity to consent) to avoid exploitation. The case below drew global attention because it raises important questions about the selection of subjects, conflict of interest when researchers have a financial stake in the products they are testing, and the extent to which IRBs should be more vigorous in overseeing research. When sued, the researchers and their institution settled the case without a trial for an undisclosed sum of money.

In 1999, an eighteen-year-old subject died in a genetics trial at one of the most prominent universities in the United States. The trial was intended to study the safety of injecting a genetically altered virus in treating ornithine transcarbamylase (OTC) deficiency. Jesse Gelsinger had a mild form of this disorder and could be managed well by diet and drugs. No one expected that he would benefit from the injection. Gelsinger developed a severe immune reaction and died four days after the injection. A year after the death the family sued the university for a variety of claims, including wrongful death.

Gelsinger's survivors alleged that researchers had improperly admitted him into the trial, as the young man had clinical findings that should have excluded him. The lawsuit also alleged that researchers had a conflict of interest because several of them had a financial stake in the product. Specifically, the lead investigator, James Wilson, had financial interests in Genovo, the private-sector biotechnology company behind the project. The suit also alleged that Gelsinger was never advised of certain adverse effects of the injection in earlier humans and animals, including deaths of monkeys.

This case, with its focus on informed consent, illustrates much of what is wrong with the work of ethics committees. On a certain view, the primary responsibility of IRBs is to ensure that informed consent is obtained. This focus obscures, however, the responsibilities of the boards to *protect from harm* and not just inform subjects about potential risks. Some people should not be offered risky interventions in the first place, and IRBs should observe that rule.

One view is that it would have been better to enroll newborn children with severe cases of this disease rather than adults. Although newborns could not consent to participate, they would be harmed less if they died because they were already at grave risk of death. A baby with a severe case of OTC deficiency and who died as a result of the intervention would not be worse off than if the trial had not occurred at all. In other words, the IRB could have chosen a pathway in which harms of death could have been minimized by requiring that the investigators use other subjects.

There probably were omissions in the consent process with Jesse Gelsinger. However, even if he had been advised of the conflicts and adverse events, he or others like him might have still agreed to enter the trial. It therefore falls to ethics committees to insist on their own evaluation of harm. In this case, would it not have been better to conduct the trial in incompetent persons (newborns) rather than with adults who face significantly greater risks, their willing assumption of risk notwithstanding?

Study Questions

1. How convincing is the notion that parents of severely affected newborns should not be asked to participate in research trials because desperation about their babies' health will not allow them to give genuinely informed consent? Even though a study is not expected to have medical benefits, might some parents not still expect medical benefit for their children?

2. Do you believe that the risks of this trial were of a magnitude that the IRB should not have allowed the study to proceed?

3. Might potential conflict of interest have undermined researchers' judgment about questions of safety when enrolling subjects?

Adapted from Julian Savelescu, "Harm, Ethics Committees, and the Gene Therapy Death," *Journal of Medical Ethics* 2001 (27): 148–150.

7.10

Genetic Warfare

Beyond alleviating disease, genetics research has many other commercial and social applications. Bioweapons involve bacterial or viral agents capable of producing disease or death. Almost by their very nature, they raise important questions about whether and to what extent they should be part of a nation's genetic research agenda.

One possible goal of biotechnology research is to design a manageable biological weapon. In 1972 the Soviet Union authorized work on "Project F" with a goal of producing a lethal virus and a vaccine. The virus could be released against enemy troops or populations, and the vaccine would protect against the return effect, namely, blowback of the virus if the wind changed direction.

Viruses or bacteria to be used in warfare might be designed in a number of ways. They might inflict near-immediate death or work more slowly. They could, for example, promote the growth of cancer or increase miscarriage, effects that would undermine an enemy population. The slow effect would have the advantage that the bioweapon would be hard to detect and trace.

It is also possible to imagine that soldiers might be genetically engineered in ways that would give advantages over the enemy. It might be possible to create transgenic soldiers with chimpanzee genes that give them greater body strength than ordinary humans. These soldiers would not be valuable in office jobs, but they might carry the day in hand-to-hand combat.

It is possible to imagine defensive uses of genetics as well. One might try to engineer a population with "pathogen countermeasures" that would protect them against engineered microbes. Of course, to detect genetic assaults and whether genetic countermeasures were effective, it would be necessary to track the genetic profiles of huge numbers of citizens. It is unclear what standard of privacy would or could prevail if this information were gathered under the umbrella of national security.

Study Questions

1. What degree of importance should be given to research in bioweapons?

2. Is there something so insidious about bioweapons that they should not be researched or used as part of any nation's military system?

Adapted from Jonathan D. Moreno, *Undue Risk: Secret State Experiments on Humans* (New York: W.H. Freeman, 2000), pp. 289–293.

Gene Transfer and the Children of Same-Sex Couples

The frontier of assisted reproductive technologies is still being mapped. It is not clear what control clinicians will have over the make-up of children they help produce through various technologies. In addition, access to assisted reproductive technologies for same-sex couples remains controversial. The case below identifies a way in which such a couple might blend their genes in a single child.

"Genome" refers to the entire genetic make-up of an organism. Gene transfer involves inserting identified genes from one genome into the genome of another organism. For the most part, human gene transfer is usually discussed as a matter of protecting against diseases and disorders; however, it is possible that it might be used to select the traits of children.

A gene might be added to an early embryonic cell that would then develop into a child bearing the trait controlled by that gene. The technique could also be used with somatic cell nuclear transfer or cloning. In this case, the somatic cell from an organism could be treated with gene transfer, and the nucleus from that cell could then be transferred to a specially treated ovum that has had its original nucleus removed. If all went right, this cell would develop into an organism that had the trait controlled by the inserted gene.

Even though there are many gay and lesbian parents, access to reproductive technologies remains politically controversial for same-sex couples and for single gay men and lesbians. It might be possible to apply gene transfer to help these couples and individuals have children. It could be used to join genetic aspects of both members of the couple in the child's genome. For example, the genes for one man's (or woman's) eye color, hair texture, and other simple traits could be inserted into a gamete that is otherwise a copy of his (or her) partner's genome. This nucleus could then be transferred into a prepared ovum, and the embryo induced to development. If this were done, the child would be genetically related to both parents.

Study Questions

1. This kind of gene transfer is hypothetical at the present time, but it is not so difficult that it must be thought of as impossible. Do you think it would be defensible for same-sex couples to use this technique to share in the genetic endowment of their children?

2. What, if any, risks of this procedure do you think would justify prohibition of the practice?

3. If this procedure carried no risks, and if it were shown to be effective and safe, would that make it more ethically acceptable?

Adapted from Timothy F. Murphy, "Entitlement to Cloning," *Cambridge Quarterly of Healthcare Ethics* 1999 (8): 364–368.

7.12

One Baby, Three Parents: Germ-Line Modification of Children

A good deal of research is done in the name of overcoming infertility. In early 2001, infertility clinicians announced that they had helped some couples conceive using the genetic endowment of three people to produce one baby. At the time of this announcement, some thirty babies around the world may have been born through the technique. This procedure is utterly new in that children are the product of three biological parents, something unprecedented in the history of the human species.

In 2001 researchers in New Jersey announced that they had helped women overcome infertility using a new technique called ooplasmic transfer, in which they transferred cytoplasm from one ovum into the ovum of a different woman. The women whose eggs received the transfer had had difficulty conceiving. The researchers hypothesized that the transfer of some cytoplasm from a healthy ovum would enhance conception and development of an embryo for women with a defect in their own eggs.

The transferred cytoplasm carries some DNA from the donor even though most of the DNA resides in the cell nucleus. The researchers say this "is the first case of human germline genetic modification resulting in normal healthy children." In carrying out this transfer, the clinicians intentionally altered the germ-line of the children. These children have, in fact, three genetic parents. They will also pass this pattern of DNA to their own children.

Study Questions

1. Because this technique produces human beings of a kind that have never existed before, should it be banned altogether?

2. What kind of risks and benefits of this technique do you think clinicians should communicate to their patients?

3. The interventions described were conducted without review and approval by an independent ethics committee. No such review is required for clinical care of individual patients. Do you think that new assisted reproductive technologies should be reviewed by an independent ethics committee before they are used in patients?

Adapted from J.A. Barritt et al., "Mitochondria in Human Offspring Derived from Ooplasmic Transplantation," *Human Reproduction* 2001 (16): 513–516; Gregory E. Kaebnick, "Inheritable Genetic Modification—It's Already Here," *Hastings Center Report* 2001 (31): 7; and Gina Kolata, "Babies Born in Experiments Have Genes from 3 People," *New York Times*, May 5, 2001.

Genetic Screening and Prenatal Diagnostics

Whereas advances in molecular biology are proceeding with breathtaking speed, it is true that the ability to identify genetic disorders far outstrips medicine's ability to treat them effectively. For many such diseases, the only treatments available are somatic (diet changes, drugs) that do not correct underlying genetic disorders. In many cases no treatments are available at all. That medicine is better at diagnosis and predicting genetic disease than at treating it raises serious questions about the value of this domain of research and how this discrepancy should be presented to the public.

"How is a successful genetics program to be defined? Much of the science involves dealing with healthy people, either carriers of single copies of recessive alleles or those suspected of bearing alleles that might affect future health. Other aspects involve the testing of those at risk of having children with genetic disease. The possibility of pregnancy termination is ineluctably part of this process, but assessing success by the number of pregnancies ended is not a satisfactory way of presenting a program's merits to the public, even though abortion reduces the incidence of disease at least as well as anti-smoking propaganda reduces lung cancer. And what of a woman found to be carrying an affected fetus who decides to continue with the pregnancy—is this to be counted as a success or a failure?

"Screening is often cost effective, at least in the starkest sense. In the Netherlands, the national genetic counseling service costs about $50 million a year. It prevents the birth of 800 to 1,600 of severely handicapped children annually. Even in that country's cost-effective health care system, the expense of lifetime care for those children would be between $500 million and $1 billion. For the United States, with a population 20 times larger (and with certain segments at higher risk because of sickle-cell disease) the figures must be multiplied many times over. To take just one example, for fragile X syndrome (a common cause of inborn mental defect) the cost of preventing a single birth is $12,000 as against the million-dollar cost of lifetime support.

"Accurate though such figures might be, they are not palatable to the public. Given that disaster, more acceptable measures of success—for example, a high proportion of families at risk of hereditary cancer being enrolled in a screening program—are called for. Escaping its negative public image is one of the biggest difficulties faced by genetics."

Study Questions

1. Is it fair to consider the reduction of the number of people with a genetic disease a success when it occurs primarily because of prenatal diagnosis and abortion?

2. In what way is it appropriate, if at all, to use calculations about the lifetime cost of care for people with genetic diseases as a means to justify prenatal genetic screening?

3. Do you agree that geneticists should represent their work to the public in a way that stresses enrollment in screening programs rather than by, say, pointing to the way in which genetic diseases have been avoided? Would morally relevant details be left out if geneticists proceeded this way?

From Steve Jones, "Genetics in Medicine: Real Promises, Unreal Expectations: One Scientist's Advice to Policymakers in the United Kingdom and the United States," *Milbank Memorial Fund,* 2000, p. 17.

Adolescents and Genetic Testing

One of the first outcomes of genetic research are diagnostic tests that allow physicians and researchers to learn whether an individual has a particular genetic trait. Testing is one thing, treatment is another. Clinical genetic medicine is in its infancy and is usually focused on testing and treatments that control the effect of genes but do not reorganize a person's genetic make-up. Increasingly, researchers are able to identify genetic traits that predict whether or not someone is likely to have disorders later in life. Whereas it is agreed that adults who are, say, forty years old should be able to test for diseases that may emerge in their fifties or later, whether younger people should also have access to predictive genetic testing is a matter of debate.

Some professional societies, such as the American Society of Human Genetics and the American College of Medical Genetics, adopted ethical advisories against some genetic testing in children. They maintain that such testing should occur only if it is important in making a diagnosis. They are otherwise opposed to genetic testing for diseases that do not emerge in childhood or that require no medical management during childhood. This prohibition is usually justified by pointing to possible harms that could result if young people knew they were likely to have disorders later in life. Younger people also might face risks of discrimination in employment and other social circumstances.

Two authors hold that this advisory is too broad. Bernice S. Elger and Timothy W. Harding maintain that the advisory treats all minors, those under the age of eighteen, as children, and a distinction should be drawn between children and adolescents age fourteen and over. In some cases, adolescents ought to have the right to genetic tests for late-onset diseases.

Adolescents often have powers to comprehend the significance of such testing, and might be harmed by *not* having access to the results. In addition, testing can be important for self-esteem and the psychological well-being of some adolescents. For example, a test might clear up worry that a young girl at age sixteen carries a gene disposing her to the breast cancer that is common in her family. The authors also hold that social discrimination has not been sufficient to justify excluding all adolescents from predictive genetic testing. On the contrary, respect for the emerging autonomy of adolescents seems to require such testing in some cases.

Study Questions

1. Why have professional organizations advised against predictive genetic testing in children?
2. What are the chief dangers to children and adolescents from these tests? How serious and how likely are these dangers?

3. What are the chief benefits that Dr. Elger and Dr. Harding see in allowing some predictive genetic testing in children fourteen years of age and older? Are you persuaded that these benefits outweigh the risks?

Adapted from Bernice S. Elger, Timothy W. Harding, "Testing Adolescents for a Hereditary Breast Cancer Gene (*BRCA1*): Respecting Their Autonomy Is in Their Best Interest," *Archives of Pediatrics and Adolescent Medicine* 2000 (154) 2: 113–119.

"Franken-Food"

Genetic alterations are useful in producing human food. Animals can be modified to produce larger amounts of products, and crops can be altered to produce greater yields or be resistant to disease. Cloning techniques are being used to produce cattle that could be used for milk and meat. Most ethical concerns associated with these developments involve the safety of humans who might eat this food and the impact of introducing genetically altered organisms into the environment.

Many animals are genetically modified to improve production and to produce new drugs. In 2002, the National Academy of Sciences issued a report warning that transgenic animals could pose food safety risks. In addition, concerns were raised about the welfare of animals produced through genetic interventions. However, the main focus of the report was on the way in which these animals might affect the environment. In particular, the government might not be ready or able to identify and prevent environmental risks coming from them.

The report referred to a genetically modified salmon as an example. This kind of salmon grows exceptionally fast. If it were approved for human consumption, it would be extremely desirable for commercial fisheries because it could be brought to market more quickly than other kinds of salmon. The report raised the possibility that this new salmon could hurt stocks of salmon in the wild. If the new salmon escaped from their breeding pens, they might displace salmon in the wild not only because they mature more quickly but also because they grow larger than most wild species. The larger size could give them significant advantage in predator-prey relationships. Most experts believe that escape to the wild by some fish is inevitable. As a way of controlling the risk, the developer of the salmon, Aqua Bounty Farms in Massachusetts, said it would create a stock that consisted entirely of sterilized females.

The FDA indicated that genetically modified animals intended for use as human food would be subject to the same regulations that govern new animal antibiotics and growth hormones. However, the report from the National Academy of Sciences raised an important legal concern: whether the FDA has the authority to deal with environmental risks of transgenic animals as against risks to humans.

The report also commented that cloned animals are on the horizon, with companies already cloning beef and dairy cattle. In 2001, the FDA ordered these animals kept from the food chain, and the director of the Center for Veterinary Medicine at the FDA said that the agency will bar cloned animals from the food supply until further research is done.

Study Questions

1. Why are moral concerns raised about introducing genetic modifications into plants and animals used as human food?

2. Dangers to the environment cannot be fully predicted when developing genetically modified organisms. Do you think this means that researchers should not modify organisms used by humans for food?

3. Are risks to the environment from genetically modified food so great that it should not be produced at all?

Adapted from Jill Carroll, Antonio Regalado, "Genetically Modified Animals May Pose Environmental Risks," *Wall Street Journal,* Aug. 21, 2002, A1.

8

Use of Animals

Introduction

One of the most famous views of animals is that of the French philosopher René Descartes (1596–1650) who saw animals as biological machines. According to a position he described in his 1637 *Discourse on Method,* animals had functions but they had no consciousness. For example, machines can emit sounds but they do not hear them; machines move but they do not know that they are moving. By analogy, Descartes maintained that animals were alive but did not have the capacity to feel. A dog might yelp if kicked, but it does not feel the pain any more than a radio winces when playing harsh music. If this view were true, human beings could use animals in painful experimentation without worry. Almost no one accepts this stark view any longer, and important moral reasons lead us to analyze the way in which researchers use animals.

Use of Animals

Dissection and other uses of animals are found in the earliest organized practices of medicine. Animals have been studied to determine their own nature and function, and for the light their anatomy and physiology can shed on those of humans. William Harvey (1578–1657) used dogs in his important studies establishing the circulation of blood. French researcher Claude Bernard (1813–1878) justified animal studies to avoid harming humans. He was convinced that humans should be spared possible harm and pain if animals could be used first to determine the effect of various interventions. As biomedical research progressed, this line of reasoning became well established in many disciplines. For example, Louis Pasteur (1822–1896) used dogs to test a vaccine against rabies.

It is an understatement to say that animals have faced distress, pain, and death in experiments. In one infamous example, researchers carried out head transplants with monkeys.[1] Military researchers used animals to study the effect of exposure to atomic blasts, microwaves, bullet injuries, burns, and so on. Chimpanzees rocketed into space well before human beings did. There is no shortage of examples.

In 1876 the United Kingdom was the first country to put laws in place dealing with animal research. Critics at the time challenged the use of animals as brutal and unnecessary, and they demanded accountability from researchers. It was in 1966 that the United States enacted its first laws in the matter.

At one end of the moral spectrum, people believe that animals have value in themselves independent of their use to human beings, and that humans should not treat animals as if they were merely means to an end. On another end, it is proposed that if alleviation of human suffering is the goal of animal experimentation, animal research is surely not the way to go. Instead, deployment of existing knowledge would do more in this regard than would development of more animal research whose benefit is confined to a select few.

The Moral Status of Animals

Important philosophical challenges are made to views that animals are merely biological machines and that humans may do anything they want with them. Indeed, the debate extends to methods used to capture, breed, confine, and kill animals. A number of salient moral issues define the terms of this debate.

Sentience and the Avoidance of Pain   Research suggests common biological foundations in anatomy and physiology between some animals and humans. Among other things, this research points to degrees of sentience and consciousness, which are the moral basis for ascribing moral interests to them. The philosophical reason for respecting animal lives, apart from human sentiment, involves the general counsel against inflicting pain where it can be avoided. Pain is pain no matter where it occurs, and animals may be used in research as long as their pain and suffering are eliminated to the extent possible.

Speciesism   One theory holds that treatment of animals is wrong in the way that sexism and racism are wrong: they are all founded on indefensible views about moral status and they lead to objectionable treatment. According to this view, it is an indefensible assumption that humans may discriminate against the interests of animals and exploit them at will. Rather, animal lives have an integrity of their own, and it is merely human arrogance to assume that their lives may be sacrificed at will. Some commentators believe that a repudiation of speciesism involves a more or less absolute prohibition against the use of animals in experimentation.[2] Whether or not this is convincing, it is generally accepted that subjecting animals to research does have to be specifically justified; it cannot be assumed that humans may treat animals in any way they wish.

Necessity   How necessary are animals to progress in biomedical research? William Paton put it this way: without animal experimentation we would still have the physics of Newton and Einstein, but we would probably not have reached the biology and medicine of Greek physician Galen.[3] By contrast, some critics maintain that most research with animals is no longer necessary because alternative methods of investigation are available. For example, students might be able to learn about frog or starfish anatomy from computer-assisted instruction rather than through dissection. Computer modeling of the influence of various infections may also bypass the need for studies of bacteria and viruses in animals. Some, however, are persuaded that biological research will continue to be necessary even if alternative methods of investigation render some uses of animals obsolete.

Corrosion of Human Values   Of concern is the belief that animal research, especially research that causes distress, harm, and death, leads to indifference and cruelty in the researchers. According to this view, the values of people who harm and kill thousands and thousands of animals in the name of research are deeply suspect. T. L. S. Sprigge insisted that killing animals because they have outlived their purpose does not cohere well with concern for them as fellow conscious subjects. This power or life and death over them does not seem compatible with respect for them as living creatures.[4] He says furthermore, readiness to treat animals as objects at the complete disposal of humans is deeply damaging to human values.

The Future of the Debate
Disagreement about the use of animals in research is manifest even among people who agree that animals are sentient, that avoidance of pain is desirable, that good moral reasons must exist for such use of animals, and that such use may not be the best way to advance knowledge. While this discussion progresses, it is also important to note the larger context of this debate. It is clear that the use of animals is under broad reconsideration on virtually every front. Some challenge ways in which animals are treated when intended as food for humans. Others object to animals being used in sport and in circuses and zoos. Closer to home for many people, animal welfarists disagree with ways in which pets are sometimes treated. They decry breeding animals

with certain traits that, while interesting to humans, are damaging to animals insofar as they open animals to ill health or disorders. It goes almost without saying that many people oppose using animals for food in that it harms animals, promotes objectionable values in humans, and is bad for the environment and human health.

In the name of biomedical science, animals have been vivisected, burned, starved, deprived of stimulation, and killed in painful ways. In the face of abuse and questionable research, it is perhaps not altogether surprising that some animal advocates commit illegal acts to draw attention to what they consider immoral uses. They have, for example, set animals free within laboratories in order to make them unuseful in further research. Most animal advocates do not commit such criminal acts, but those who do raise interesting moral questions about the scope of civil disobedience committed for their cause.

Because of such illegal actions, institutions using animals for research have stepped up their security measures and, it must be said, increased the attention given to the care of animals. Most countries now have legal standards that govern animal research, although they do not all require the same treatment. In the United States, the federal Animal Welfare Act is a cornerstone, and institutions conducting research with animals have committees that oversee experimentation. These committees follow procedures outlined in federal policy with regard to obtaining, housing, and experimenting with many animals; however, it is still a matter of debate just exactly what animals should be protected.

It appears clear that at a moral minimum, animals must be protected under a standard of beneficence, and that their capacities to feel pain, to thrive in certain environments, and to show affection should help guide decisions about their treatment.[5] It is also certain that justifications for the use of animals must become more sophisticated if researchers are to meet the pointed criticisms directed at callous and unnecessary uses.

References

1. R. Ryder, *Victims of Science* (London: Davis-Poynter, 1975).

2. See Tom Regan, *The Case for Animal Rights* (Berkeley: University of California Press, 1985); and Tom Regan, *Defending Animal Rights* (Urbana: University of Illinois Press, 2001). See also Tom Regan, Peter Singer, eds., *Animal Rights and Human Obligations* (New York: Prentice, 1976); and Peter Singer, *Animal Liberation* (New York: Ecco Press, 2001).

3. Quoted in T. L. S. Sprigge, "Animal Experimentation in Biomedical Research: A Critique," in Raanan Gillon, ed., *Principles of Healthcare Ethics* (Chichester: John Wiley & Sons, 1994), pp. 1053–1065.

4. Sprigge.

5. Tristam H. Engelhardt, Jr., *The Foundations of Bioethics*, 2nd ed. (New York: Oxford University Press, 1996), pp. 145–146.

8.1

Animal Entrapment

Although scientists agree on the need to study animal specimens, that does not mean that specimens can be collected in any manner whatsoever. The case below raises interesting questions about the need for particular specimens, ways they are collected, and differences between the letter and the spirit of legal regulations.

In 1992, John Trochet, a University of California graduate student in ornithology, identified a yellow-green vireo at Carlsbad Caverns National Park in New Mexico. This was the northernmost sighting of this bird, which is indigenous to a region ranging throughout Central America, but is not usually found north of Mexico. Although the bird had been sighted in southern Texas and Arizona, it had never been seen at this latitude. The bird may have migrated north seeking new territory because of loss of habitat, it may have lost its way, or it may have been blown off course in a storm. It might even have been transported and released by a traveler. Scientists who were interested to see this bird outside its usual habitat and bird-watching enthusiasts gathered to watch the vireo. They wondered if it was the same one that had been reported in the area the year before.

It is a violation of federal law to collect animals in national parks. Knowing this, Trochet made a tape recording of the bird's song. When birds hear these tapes played, they think it is another bird and follow to investigate. Trochet did not want to wait to see if the bird would fly off park property: it might not leave the park, or he might not be able to capture it even if it did. Instead, Trochet used the song to lure the bird out of the park. Once the vireo followed the recorded song and left national park property, Trochet caught it in a net and suffocated it by holding it in a tight fist. He had a license to take specimens in this way, as long as he did not do it on federal land. When the bird was dead, Trochet sent the specimen back to the museum of ornithology at the University of California. Local bird watchers learned what he had done and were outraged.

Study Questions

1. What argument can be offered that it was important to have this particular bird as a research specimen for the ornithology museum? Could the researcher not have obtained a specimen from a location where the bird is more plentiful?

2. Was Trochet's method of capturing and killing this bird objectionable in any way?

Adapted from F. Barbara Orlans, Tom L. Beauchamp, Rebecca Dresser, David B. Morton, John P. Gluck, *The Human Use of Animals: Case Studies in Ethical Choice* (New York: Oxford University Press, 1998), pp. 191–205, especially 191–195.

The Study of Animal Aggression

The study of animal behavior that harms others animals is interesting in its own right and because it may have implications for human aggression. The following case raises questions about appropriate ways of studying animal aggression. First among those questions is the way in which the artificial environment of the laboratory may contribute to such behavior. Beyond that, it is worth while to examine justifications for subjecting animals to harm and to find ways to reduce it.

In a 1984 article in the journal *Animal Behavior,* two Northern Ireland scientists, Robert W. Elwood and Malcomb C. Ostenmeyer, reported their findings on factors that influence adult male rodents to kill young of their own species. Various hypotheses exist on why they do this, but presumably it gives them an advantage in perpetuating their own genes.

Elwood and Ostenmeyer wanted to know whether they could identify factors that promoted or inhibited this behavior. It had been suggested that copulation with a female mouse was an inhibitor, and the two men tested this hypothesis. They put sexually naive (never mated) adult male mice alone in cages and introduced live newborns into those cages. They identified mice that repeatedly killed the infants and used them in a series of experiments. Males that ignored the newborns were not used for further study.

The researchers introduced killer mice to females for copulation and tested the males for infanticidal behavior on three occasions: before the experiment, on the day of copulation, and eighteen days after copulation. Copulation by itself did not inhibit the males from killing young mice placed into the cage. However, if the males were allowed to cohabit with females, they were less inclined to that behavior. During the entire study, the adult males killed eighty-seven newborn mice.

In a companion editorial on the study, the ethics committee of the journal noted that the young mice were killed instantaneously and did not suffer.

Study Questions

1. How important do you believe this kind of scientific study is? Given the large number of mice used in research settings, is it not true that this study could provide important information to many researchers?

2. What, if anything, is ethically problematic about this study?

3. What other methods, if any, might have been used to achieve results without exposing so many mice to death?

Adapted from F. Barbara Orlans, Tom L. Beauchamp, Rebecca Dresser, David B. Morton, John P. Gluck, *The Human Use of Animals: Case Studies in Ethical Choices* (New York: Oxford University Press, 1998), pp. 155–170, especially 157–158.

8.3

Baboon Head Injury Experiments

The use of animals in research becomes ethically problematic when it involves highly intelligent species. Although a good deal of knowledge can be obtained from primate models of human disorders, the extent to which these animals should be subjected to research is a source of continuing controversy. This case raises questions not only about the proper use of primates and the appropriate degree of oversight, but also about the ethics of animal welfarists who violate the law.

In the early 1980s, Thomas A. Gennarelli, a professor at the University of Pennsylvania, was studying the effect of head injuries in baboons. His goal was to identify an animal model in which to study physiological and anatomical effects of head trauma in humans.

Baboons were first treated with PCP, a dissociative drug also known as angel dust, to make them easier to restrain. They were then treated with nitrous oxide, but this drug was withdrawn up to one hour before the intervention, because the animals had to be conscious just before the injury and general anesthesia would have rendered some of the tests meaningless. The researchers said they would administer more nitrous oxide if the experiment went "awry."

The animals were strapped to tables and fitted with monitors, and their heads were cemented inside a helmet. A hydraulic piston then suddenly twisted or jolted their heads. This device could simulate 2,000 times the force of gravity. The monkeys were typically comatose and paralyzed after the intervention, although some died. The surviving animals were sustained for two months, at which point they were sacrificed and the effect of the injuries on their brains was studied.

In May 1984, members of the Animal Liberation Front (ALF) invaded Gennarelli's laboratory, stole videotapes of the experiments, and released them to the public. People for the Ethical Treatment of Animals (PETA) released an edited version of the tapes, showing the injured and distressed monkeys.

After its first raid, ALF made two other raids, this time stealing thirteen animals from the University of Pennsylvania veterinary school. In the public outcry that followed, the adequacy of anesthesia was questioned, as was the general treatment of the baboons. The validity of the scientific hypothesis underlying the research was also criticized. Animal welfarists conducted sit-ins at the National Institutes of Health, which was funding Gennarelli's research. In direct response to this case, Congress enacted new laws mandating more rigorous oversight of laboratory animals.

Study Questions

1. What ethical issues, if any, are associated with intentional administration of head injuries to baboons?

2. How important is it that results from these studies can be used to help protect and treat human beings who suffer parallel injuries?

3. Civil disobedience involves intentional violations of the law to draw attention to unethical policy or behavior. Do you believe that thefts of laboratory animals can be considered civil disobedience?

Adapted from F. Barbara Orlans, Tom L. Beauchamp, Rebecca Dresser, David B. Morton, John P. Gluck, *The Human Use of Animals: Case Studies in Ethical Choices* (New York: Oxford University Press, 1998), pp. 71–87, especially 71–73.

Animal-to-Human Xenografts

Physicians are often interested in clinical innovations that might extend the life of patients with no other means of treatment, such as those with major organ failure. Not only is there a daunting lack of available organs for transplantation, not all patients are candidates for the procedure. In one case, physicians proposed the transplantation of a baboon's liver into a human. Tissues transplanted from other species to humans are known as xenografts. The case raises significant questions about the merits of transplantation with a great degree of unknown risk, such as the possibility of introducing animal viruses into humans.

A thirty-five-year-old man lapsed into a coma after his liver was destroyed by hepatitis B infection. A liver transplant was necessary or the man would die, but physicians believed that the hepatitis virus would destroy a new liver as well. Moreover, the man was also infected with HIV, making him already at severe risk of immunosuppression. After transplantation, patients must take certain drugs to suppress the immune system to ward off rejection.

Shortly after the man lapsed into a coma, his physicians replaced his liver with a liver taken from a fifteen-year-old male baboon. The patient had previously provided consent for the surgery. It was believed that the baboon's liver would be resistant to the pathogenic activity of the hepatitis infection.

For a short time the man's health improved substantially, so that five days after receiving the animal's liver he could eat and walk. In fact, the liver grew to the size of the human organ. This success was short lived, however. The patient lapsed into renal failure and experienced several infections that were difficult to treat. He developed jaundice, and about two and one-half months after the operation he died. Liver failure did not appear to be the immediate cause of death, but immunological rejection of the organ might have been a contributing cause.

The surgeon overseeing the case, Thomas Starzl, nevertheless predicted that this kind of xenograft would eventually be successful. The intervention provoked criticism that science had not yet shown that such transplantation could work, especially with regard to the liver's ability to function in a human in the long term. Meanwhile, animal welfarists protested the use of baboons as a source of spare parts.

Study Questions

1. Given that he was facing death, the patient consented to receiving a baboon liver. Was his desperate condition a reason to worry whether or not he genuinely understood the risks of a cross-species transplantation? What risks and benefits do you believe should be communicated to a patient who would undergo such a procedure?

2. Do you believe it is an appropriate use of medical resources to try and rescue patients with expensive and unproved treatments? Or should these patients be offered palliative care instead?

3. How convincing is the view that baboons should not be killed to use their organs for medical treatment of human beings?

Adapted from F. Barbara Orlans, Tom L. Beauchamp, Rebecca Dresser, David B. Morton, John P. Gluck, *The Human Use of Animals: Case Studies in Ethical Choice* (New York: Oxford University Press, 1998), pp. 55–69, especially 55–57.

8.5

Kitten Experiments

Animal welfarists have used various techniques to investigate research and sway the public about the ethics of animal experimentation. They conduct undercover videotaping of animal research, report on research activities, and carry out public protests. While such efforts are accepted methods of protest and social change, questions remain about these groups' investigations: are they thorough and unbiased enough to provide a basis for balanced decisions? Indirectly, the case here raises questions about the responsibilities of researchers to institute mechanisms for educating the public about the nature and value of their research.

In 1995, PETA began an undercover investigation at the Boys Town National Research Hospital, a Catholic-sponsored institution in Omaha, Nebraska, and revealed their findings at a news conference in Omaha in 1996. According to PETA, the hospital carried out experiments in which kittens had their heads sliced open and their nerves severed to study deafness.

A variety of protests ensued, including dumping used kitty litter at offices of the hospital and occupying Boys Town's offices. One picketer, dressed as the devil, climbed onto the roof and declared "Satan Loves Boys Town Cat Experiments." Several deaf activists joined in the protests.

An administrator for PETA, Mary Beth Sweetland, said, "We have offered to place the surviving cats, and we appeal to Boys Town to please not use mice, guinea pigs, or rats, who suffer every bit as much pain as kittens. We urge Boys Town to concentrate on bringing joy to children rather than ever again hurting animals." In 1997, Brigitte Bardot, actress, animal rights activist, and Catholic, joined forces with PETA, asking Pope John Paul II to help halt the kitten experiments at Boys Town. Bardot sent the Pope a PETA videotape said to show the kittens' suffering, and faxed copies of her letter to regional Boys Town offices across the United States.

A short time later, Boys Town announced that kittens would no longer be used in tests. At that time, PETA pointed out that Boys Town had originally claimed that kittens were indispensable to their deafness studies.

Study Questions

1. Is it convincing that animals should not be used for experiments if similar information might be obtained by using computer models or historical data? Should researchers assume a moral prohibition against killing animals in experiments unless they must absolutely do so to obtain important information?

2. As told from the perspective of PETA, researchers appear to have bowed to negative publicity. Do you think that activism can improve research?

Adapted from www.peta-online.org. Downloaded June 21, 2000.

Depriving Primates of Mothers

In the case below, monkeys were taken from their mothers and housed with inanimate mother surrogates in order to study their development. Researchers wanted to know which elements of attachment to the mother were most important in monkey development. By all accounts, this research was extremely influential in its time.

Harry F. Harlow wanted to study the mechanisms by which newborn rhesus monkeys bond to their mothers. These infants are highly dependent on their mothers for nutrition, protection, comfort, and socialization. What exactly, though, was the basis of the bond? Was it primarily a matter of nutrition, a function of an innate suckling instinct, an innate need to touch and to cling, or something else? These questions have parallels in human development, and Harlow thought primate development might shed some light on them.

To examine the nature of infant attachment to its mother, Harlow removed eight monkeys from their mothers immediately after birth and placed them in cages with access to two mother surrogates. One mother surrogate was constructed from wood and covered with terrycloth, and the second was constructed of wire. The baby monkeys nursed from bottles hidden in the surrogates, four from the cloth surrogate and four from the wire surrogate. A heating pad in a neutral part of the cage was also available to the infants.

The animals were studied for 165 days. Most preferred to spend time with the cloth surrogate no matter how they obtained their feedings. Harlow took the findings to mean that a nutritional theory of attachment was insufficient to explain the nature of bonding by the infant rhesus to its mother. He further tested this by introducing challenges to the monkeys that would provoke fear. In these challenges, the infant monkeys took refuge with the cloth monkey. Other studies seemed to confirm the importance of the cloth surrogate—but not the wire surrogate—to the monkeys.

Study Questions

1. How important do you think the research objectives of this study were? Were the consequences for the monkeys balanced by a comparable gain in knowledge?

2. The social fate of these animals is an ethical concern, as this study might have left the monkeys socially stunted in ways that limited their well-being. How might the researchers have tried to control such stunting?

3. Many people believe that data from unethical research in humans should not be used. If this research with monkeys was unethical, would it be defensible to apply the same standard here: that unethically obtained results should not be applied further?

Adapted from F. Barbara Orlans, Tom L. Beauchamp, Rebecca Dresser, David B. Morton, John P. Gluck, *The Human Use of Animals: Case Studies in Ethical Choices* (New York: Oxford University Press, 1998), pp. 171–187, especially 173–177.

The Green Fluorescent Rabbit

One of the most unexpected applications of genetic science has been in the art world. So far, only a few artists have used genetic technologies, but it is likely that this use will increase. This case raises questions about the limits to which biological organisms may be modified for artistic purposes. It also raises questions about whether limits should be placed on the way in which the public produces genetically modified organisms. From the artist's point of view, production of new organisms also raises questions about the place of genetics in everyday life and its role in social criticism.

In 2000, Eduardo Kac, a professor at the School of the Art Institute in Chicago, relying on the help of French researchers, injected a gene for green fluorescent protein into a rabbit zygote. The gene was taken from jellyfish that exhibit a green fluorescence. The zygote was implanted into a rabbit uterus where it developed to birth. Under the right fluorescent light, the adult rabbit's fur glows green.

Kac did this, he claims, to stimulate debate about the uses of biotechnology. He exhibited the rabbit at various venues in hope of showing how biotechnologies are creeping into our lives. Some animal activists objected to his use of the rabbit. Others wonder whether this animal can be considered "art."

Not resting on his laurels, Kac translated a Biblical passage into a gene sequence using a series of substitutions between letters and DNA sequences. The passage in question was "Let man have dominion over the fish of the sea, and over the fowl of the air, and over every living thing that moves upon the earth." He then inserted the gene sequence into bacteria grown in a petri dish. He made arrangements for Internet users to be able to flash ultraviolet lights on the petri dish, causing the gene sequence to mutate. Kac claimed that his piece showed how easy it is to manipulate genes, with no questions asked by anybody.

Study Questions

1. Many transgenic animals (animals with genes from two species) are used in laboratory research. The one in this case was produced without regulatory oversight. What ethical concerns are associated with private individuals producing transgenic animals?

2. Is it desirable to use art such as this transgenic rabbit to promote discussion and attention to the way in which genetics can infiltrate and change human lives? Was this purpose "serious" enough to justify producing the rabbit?

Adapted from Lori Andrews, "Weird Science," *Chicago Magazine*, Aug. 2000, pp. 22–23. See also ekac.org.

Animal Vivisection

Many animal welfarists believe that animals are misused in research. The statement below, from PETA, raises a number of arguments against vivisection. These should be examined individually and as a whole to determine whether they make a definitive case against using live animals in research.

"There are many reasons to oppose vivisection. For example, enormous physiological variations exist among rats, rabbits, dogs, pigs, and human beings. A 1989 study to determine the carcinogenicity of fluoride illustrated this fact. Approximately 520 rats and 520 mice were given daily doses of the mineral for two years. Not one mouse was adversely affected by the fluoride, but the rats experienced health problems including cancer of the mouth and bone. As test data cannot accurately be extrapolated from a mouse to a rat, it can't be argued that data can accurately be extrapolated from either species to a human.

"In many cases, animal studies do not just hurt animals and waste money; they harm and kill people, too. The drugs thalidomide, Zomax, and DES were all tested on animals and judged safe but had devastating consequences for the humans who used them. A General Accounting Office report, released in May 1990, found that more than half of the prescription drugs approved by the Food and Drug Administration between 1976 and 1985 caused side effects that were serious enough to cause the drugs to be withdrawn from the market or relabeled. All of these drugs had been tested on animals.

"Animal experimentation also misleads researchers in their studies. Dr. Albert Sabin, who developed the oral polio vaccine, cited in testimony at a congressional hearing this example of the dangers of animal-based research: 'Paralytic polio could be dealt with only by preventing the irreversible destruction of the large number of motor nerve cells, and the work on prevention was delayed by an erroneous conception of the nature of the human disease based on misleading experimental models of the disease in monkeys.' And tax dollars would be better spent preventing human suffering in the first place through education programs and medical assistance programs for low-income individuals—helping the more than 30 million US citizens who cannot afford health insurance—rather than making animals sick.

"Most killer diseases in this country (heart disease, cancer, and stroke) can be prevented by eating a low-fat, vegetarian diet, refraining from smoking and alcohol abuse, and exercising regularly. These simple lifestyle changes can also help prevent arthritis, adult-onset diabetes, ulcers, and a long list of other illnesses. It is not surprising that those who make money experimenting on animals or supplying vivisectors with cages, restraining devices, food for caged animals (like the Lab Chow made by Purina Mills), and tiny guillotines to destroy animals whose lives are no longer considered useful insist that nearly every medical advance has been made through the use of animals. Although every drug and procedure must now be tested on animals before hitting the market, this does not mean that animal studies are invaluable, irreplaceable, or even of minor importance or that alternative methods could not have been used."

Study Questions

1. How convincing is the position that animals should not be used for research since variations among species will confound the value of this research?

2. How convincing is it to say that much animal research is wasteful and harmful because its results do not always extend to human beings?

3. Is it true that research with animals tends to promote health interventions that are less effective than other means of protecting health? How might this be known to be true or false?

Downloaded with minor stylistic changes from www.PETA.com, July 22, 2000.

Primate Language Acquisition

The use of higher primates in research is debated because of concerns about their intelligence and moral status. An associated question is how they are treated after the research is over. The case below raises many key ethical questions.

R. Alen and Beatrix T. Gardiner acquired a young female chimpanzee, named Washoe, to test its ability to acquire American Sign Language (ASL), which is used by the deaf. Earlier attempts in instruction had not been successful, but the Gardiners wanted to study the extent to which the animal might learn signs and gestures. The Gardiners taught the chimp as parents might teach human children: to use human utensils while eating, to dress, to play with toys, and to use the toilet. Washoe was given considerable human attention and did not interact with other chimpanzees. The Gardiners used ASL in front of her as much as possible. By the time Washoe was about four years old, she was able to use approximately 132 signs.

At five years of age Washoe was moved to the Institute for Primate Studies at the University of Oklahoma, where she was introduced to other chimps who had been taught to sign. The goal was to determine whether the chimps used signs when communicating among themselves, which they did to some extent.

Eventually Washoe delivered a baby, but it died. Shortly afterward, she was given the baby of another chimp to see whether she would teach it to sign. The researchers made sure never to sign in front of the baby, but Washoe and the other chimps did. Eventually, the baby acquired approximately fifty-one signs.

Washoe and her baby were later moved to another housing facility at Central Washington University where they joined three other signing chimpanzees the Gardiners had raised. The animals continue to be used in observational and noninvasive studies for language and behavior. Other signing chimpanzees were ultimately sent to biomedical research facilities or wildlife centers where little or no attention was given to their abilities to communicate.

Study Questions

1. What exactly is the nature of deprivation faced by chimpanzees if they leave a signing environment, and why is it thought to be morally significant?

2. Before teaching chimpanzees higher-order skills, do researchers have an obligation to ensure that the animals will remain in an enriched environment? Should researchers not teach chimpanzees signing if they cannot be kept in an environment that will encourage and use it?

Adapted from F. Barbara Orlans, Tom L. Beauchamp, Rebecca Dresser, David B. Morton, John P. Gluck, *The Human Use of Animals: Case Studies in Ethical Choices* (New York: Oxford University Press, 1998), pp. 139–154, especially 139–142.

8.10

Whale Research

International conventions forbid the killing of various kinds of whales in order to protect them from extinction. This prohibition causes conflicts when exceptions to the rule seem to be exploited as pretexts. The case below involves the use of whales as food, even when they are killed in the name of research. A key question is whether legitimate scientific purposes are involved in hunting whales, or whether the exception that permits hunting is being used as a cover to provide a traditional food.

In August 2000, Japanese researchers announced that they would kill about fifty Bryde's whales and ten sperm whales to carry out various research projects. Hunting these whales has been prohibited since 1986 except for scientific purposes. Critics of this hunt immediately claimed that the research was a thinly disguised effort to produce food. Whale meat is a traditional food in Japan, and after research is completed, the whales are sold for food. In fact, the research unit brings in about $35 million per year from these sales.

Members of the International Whaling Commission objected, claiming that the studies could be conducted without killing. They suggested that nonlethal biopsy darts could be used to retrieve small tissue samples for analysis. However, the director of the Japanese Cetacean Research Institute said that studies of internal organs and stomach contents could not progress unless the animals were captured and killed. Some Japanese commentators suggested that prejudice against traditional foods was the real motive for banning whale hunting and objected to this cultural imperialism.

Study Questions

1. To what extent may cultural imperialism (in this case, distaste on the part of most of the world at eating whales) play a role in objections to Japanese whaling?
2. Are you convinced that whales must be killed in order to conduct research?

Calvin Sims, "Japan, Feasting on Whale, Sniffs at 'Culinary Imperialism' of U.S.," *New York Times,* Aug. 10, 2000, pp. A1, A8.

Public Access to Animal Research Review Committees

The late twentieth century saw considerable growth in the number of public groups objecting to many, if not all, animal experiments. One way that groups seek to influence and perhaps eliminate this practice is through access to animal research review committees. These committees have a legal responsibility to ensure that animals are housed and fed appropriately, that pain is minimized during the course of experimentation, and that animals are humanely killed when death is appropriate to the experiment. They also have the right to approve or disapprove research. Researchers and animal welfare groups often disagree about the extent to which these committees should be open to the public.

In the 1980s, the Progressive Animal Welfare Society (PAWS) brought several suits against the University of Washington in Seattle to gain access to meetings and documents of the animal research committee. Like many universities of its stature, the University of Washington uses tens of thousands of animals in research each year. PAWS claimed the state's so-called Sunshine Laws required the university to open its committee meetings to the public. Such laws are intended to open the operations of government to public scrutiny and participation.

The courts held that the university should open these meetings to the public, and in doing so, set aside a considerable number of the university's objections. The university was concerned that certain animal welfare groups were likely to introduce difficulties with experiments already under way, and also feared confrontation in public protests.

Another alllegation was that opening meetings to the public could lead to exposure of scientific ideas that could be used by competitors. The overall result would make the university a less competitive place to conduct research, which would affect not only researchers pursuing funding but also the quality of education in general. Most dramatically, the university worried that opening meetings might endanger researchers, pointing to several instances in which researchers had been picketed at their homes and received death threats.

Study Questions

1. Why would animal welfarists try to gain access to committee meetings that review studies involving animals?

2. Given that animal welfarists would have no say over whether or not studies were carried out—they would have no voting privileges—why would a university wish to keep them from meetings?

3. How valid are concerns that closed meetings are necessary to protect intellectual property, the decorum of meetings, and maybe even the lives of researchers?

Adapted from F. Barbara Orlans, Tom L. Beauchamp, Rebecca Dresser, David B. Morton, John P. Gluck, *The Human Use of Animals: Case Studies in Ethical Choices* (New York: Oxford University Press, 1998), pp. 103–117, especially 105–107.

8.12

___

Saving the Florida Panther

Where there are no conflicts, there are no ethical dilemmas. In the case below, the dilemma is between maintaining an animal in the wild and developing land for human use. Certain methods could be used to try to save the animal's habitat, but it is unclear whether they would work. If the conservation efforts were inexpensive and did not dislocate other projects, there would be no difficulty; but they are expensive, politically difficult, and conflict with other options.

The Florida panther is one of fifteen recognized subspecies of the North American mountain lion. It once ranged from eastern Texas to South Carolina, but now exists in the wild only in remote parts of southern Florida. The animal is medium-sized and golden-brown; it has stiff hair, a distinctive crook in its tail, a whorl of hair on its back, and irregular white flecking on and around its head. A 1989 report indicated that as few as forty of these animals may be left in the state. Between 1980 and 1986, ten panthers were killed on state highways. One estimate suggested that the animal could be extinct in the wild within twenty years.

Efforts to sustain the panthers in the wild face considerable obstacles. It is not known, for example, how many animals would be necessary to maintain a viable population. In addition, genetic inbreeding may doom the animal; studies of sperm revealed increased abnormalities over the years. The land necessary for prey is also dwindling because of encroaching human development.

Adult panthers eat as much as a deer a week, or the equivalent amount of boar; pregnant panthers may require two deer a week. To sustain this amount of prey, one biologist suggested that a population of fifty animals would require a set-aside of nearly three million acres. It would be difficult, however, to find a single land area of that size. Another biologist proposed having several smaller plots connected by land corridors. Others reject both these solutions, seeing them as politically impossible and unlikely to work. They believe the costs of trying to save the panther in the wild in Florida are too high, and efforts should be focused on preserving the animals in zoos or similar institutions.

Kristin Shrader-Frechette, a philosopher who has studied issues in ecology, maintains that conserving this animal is justified because it will benefit everybody, both in the present and the future. In addition, conservation takes priority over human development of the land, because development benefits only a few. She also notes that development carries a lot of unwanted costs. Conservation might also incorporate wildlife recreation projects to accommodate human interests in these wildlife refuges. Therefore, people who do not want to save the panther in the wild have the burden of proof to show that their proposals are authentic indicators of welfare for present and future generations.

Study Questions

1. What is the main reason for setting aside a significant habitat for this animal?

2. Why is setting aside habitat for this animal supposed to be an authentic indicator of welfare for present and future generations?

3. Is it really the case that developing land benefits only a few individuals whereas using land for panther habitat serves a larger benefit?

4. Are other mechanisms, such as cloning, possible by which this animal might be preserved? If so, do they undercut the need for a land set-aside?

Adapted from Kristin Shrader-Frechette, *Ethics of Scientific Research* (Lanham, MD: Rowman & Littlefield, 1994), pp. 119–138.

8.13

Expanding the Animal Welfare Act

For a variety of reasons, mice, rats, and birds were excluded from key federal legislation that governs the use of animals in research. As a result, private researchers may use those animals in ways that might not conform to provisions required for other animals. Some maintain that because of voluntary ways of protecting animal welfare, and because of the sheer number of animals involved, it would be a mistake to include mice, rats, and birds under the Animal Welfare Act.

The Animal Welfare Act of 1985 requires particular kinds of treatment for a variety of animals being used in research: primates, dogs, cats, rabbits, gerbils, and others. Researchers who use these species must register with the United States Department of Agriculture (USDA) and be open to inspection by representatives of that agency. They must comply with a variety of provisions intended to promote humane treatment of animals. At minimum, pain and distress must be minimized.

This statute excludes, however, species used in almost 90 percent of United States research: rats, mice, and birds. The United States is probably the largest user of research animals in the world. Yet it is the only country to exclude these animals from protection laws. "Their exclusion leaves significant loopholes in the law's effectiveness and is detrimental to the excluded animals' welfare."

Mice and rats are as capable of perceiving pain as other animals covered by legislation; in fact, their perception of pain resembles that of humans. Birds' perception of pain is well recognized. It is problematic then that privately funded organizations and some private colleges use these animals in ways that run counter to legislation. Biotechnology companies, for example, engineer mice to simulate human diseases (diabetes, cancer, multiple sclerosis, arthritis, etc.). These animals experience chronic pain, weakened body parts, physical abnormalities, and more.

Extending the Animal Welfare Act to these species would promote the three Rs: (1) refinement of techniques so as to minimize or eliminate pain in animals, (2) reduction of the total number of animals used in research, and (3) replacement of animals to the extent possible with nonanimal alternatives.

Many believe that extending the Act is not necessary because other provisions protect and promote animal welfare, and thus it would not improve their welfare. Moreover, some institutions pursue voluntary policies of animal welfare. Against this argument, it is to be said that the USDA has mechanisms of oversight and monitoring that are not available to other agencies. To be sure, the department would require more money to include these species under its domain, but "Unless action is taken now by U.S.D.A., the biotechnology industry may well grow beyond control, and the welfare of many animals will suffer immeasurably."

Study Questions

1. What is the most important ethical reason for extending the Animal Welfare Act to rats, mice, and birds? How convincing is it?

2. To what extent is it morally persuasive that rats, mice, and birds are different enough not to require the same legal provisions for their welfare as other animals?

3. To what extent do practical considerations (e.g., burden on the oversight agency) justify or not justify extending the provisions of the Animal Welfare Act to widely used research animals?

Adapted from F. Barbara Orlans, "The Injustice of Excluding Laboratory Rats, Mice, and Birds from the Animal Welfare Act," *Kennedy Institute of Ethics Journal* 2000 (10): 229–238.

8.14

Cloning Pets

Since 1997, researchers have cloned sheep, mice, cows, goats, and other mammals. The case below raises certain ethical questions associated with the cloning of the familiar family pet.

In 1998, an anonymous donor gave Texas A & M University $2.4 million to clone a beloved dog, Missy. Additional donations brought the total to well over $3 million. A researcher there, Lou Hawthorne, subsequently set up a private corporation for pet cloning: Genetic Savings and Clone. Hawthorne claims that people want to clone their pets because they love them and want them around forever. Many pets have been neutered, and therefore could not be genetic parents. Moreover, many owners of mixed-breed dogs want to clone their dogs because their unique genetics can't be duplicated through breeding. Movie and television companies would like cloned animals so they could use more than one identical animal: even dogs need a break in Hollywood.

Animals can't be duplicated, however. Hawthorne warns his clients, "You aren't going to get the same animal with the same bond. Your bond with your animal is not clonable." Nicholas Dodman, director of animal behavior at Tufts University School of Veterinary Medicine also noted, "No matter how hard you plan it, you couldn't raise the dog under identical circumstances." The clone would be a blank slate, having none of the original dog's experiences.

Right now, no company clones dogs or cats, but several take tissue samples from the mouth and abdomen. Cells are cultured and frozen in the expectation that the material can be used for cloning in the future. Because of concerns about the aging process in clones, biotech companies recommend taking samples from young and healthy animals, but a veterinarian could also take a sample from an animal immediately after its death.

During the tissue sampling, some animals may need to be forcibly held down or require an anesthetic. The American Veterinary Medical Association has issued no advisory about cloning, but Michael Fox, senior scholar of bioethics at the Humane Society of the United States, thinks the process exploits female dogs: "You're going to need a lot of females to produce ova, then another batch to receive the clones. Female dogs come into heat only twice a year. You can't be waiting for all these dogs, so there is going to be hormonal manipulation to ovulate." He continues: "If people want a dog like the one they had, go adopt one from an animal shelter. If you loved one dog, why can't you love all dogs? Put the hundreds of thousands of dollars into helping dogs in your community and around the world."

Study Questions

1. What is the relative importance of trying to discover a way to clone pets?

2. Is there anything morally problematic about accepting tissue samples for cloning when there is no commercially proven technique for doing so?

3. Are any of the foreseen consequences of this project so damaging—to female dogs kept for breeding, to dogs left unadopted—that researchers should not pursue cloning in this area?

Adapted from Ellen Kanner, "Welcome to the Clone Age," *Dog Fancy*, August 2000, pp. 26–30. See also www.missyplicity.com.

9

Authorship and Publication

Introduction

At first blush it might seem that authorship and publication are the least problematic aspects of scientific research. In fact, they trigger many important ethical questions. Authorship and publication are not neutral parts of the scientific process. Writing and presenting research to the scientific community, to physicians, and to the public involve ethical issues that are central to the integrity of science. Fraud and misrepresentation are antithetical to the basic goals of scientific research: they obstruct the very purposes of research. Other kinds of misconduct such as misattributed authorship and plagiarism may not involve falsified data or dubious interpretations, but they distort relationships within the scientific community and the relationship of researchers to the public.

Fraud and Misrepresentation
Fraud, fabrication, and plagiarism are probably the best known forms of research misconduct. Fraud and fabrication involve willful misrepresentation of

data: inaccurate reports, manipulations of actual findings, or presentation of data that were never produced by the study.[1] Plagiarism, a word derived from the Latin for kidnapping, involves the appropriation of another's work as one's own without the real author's permission or attribution.

In a number of clear cases researchers simply invented data or misrepresented actual data in extreme ways; however, it is not always easy to distinguish fraud from fact. One 1990s case that garnered national attention involved accusations that Teresa Imanishi-Kari and her colleagues falsified data published in the prestigious journal *Cell*.[2] An employee in her laboratory initiated a series of accusations that turned on data, laboratory records, and tests that were highly technical and difficult to interpret. The National Institutes of Health eventually conducted several investigations in which Dr. Imanishi-Kari was found guilty of reporting fraudulent data. In response, Dr. Imanishi-Kari filed suit against the investigators and was exonerated in court of wrongdoing. Indeed, it appears that some of the findings originally used to establish her guilt were flawed in the extreme. Despite being cleared in court, the investigations derailed this scientist from her work and diminished her stature in the scientific community, not to mention the considerable expenses she incurred in defending herself from the accusations.

The extent to which fraud, fabrication, and plagiarism find their way into published journals is not well studied. Some contend that these are comparatively minor problems because of the scientific commitment to replication of studies. These commentators expect that no such material will stand unchallenged for very long because it is a tenet of the scientific method to examine the methods and conclusions of other scientists. Thus, in the fullness of time all error and fraud will be rooted out because science is by its very nature self-correcting. Others agree that scientific investigation will eventually uncover all fraud, fabrication, and misconduct, but they note that these misdeeds have real and objectionable consequences. This is especially true for the clinical sciences in which study findings are applied to the care of patients. Because of these consequences, many scientists urge measures to prevent misconduct before it occurs, to spare expense, time, reputations, and harm to patients.

Editorial Review and Decisions to Publish

The amount of fraud, fabrication, and plagiarism might be reduced if scientific reports mattered less than they do. Researchers have *many* incentives to publish and to do so in the most prestigious journals. Success in academic settings is often governed by the infamous doctrine of publish or perish. Each field has key journals that are deemed to be the most important; researchers who write books submit their work to a few elite university presses. The pressure to publish and to publish in the most prestigious and influential places can create emotional dissonance.

An important way in which publishers can work against fraud, fabrication, and plagiarism is also the key way in which they can ensure the value and integrity of the science in question: peer review. Most journals and university presses evaluate the merits of a study through editorial evaluation and reviews solicited from knowledgeable experts in the field. These experts are asked to offer their anonymous opinions on the validity of the work. This review not only holds scientific findings up to scrutiny, it also gives independent reviewers the opportunity to alert journals to misconduct and allows them to make suggestions about improving the work.

Journals may blind an article when they send it to reviewers; that is, they withhold certain information that could identify the authors of the study. In addition to authors' names, they may withhold other information, such as where the study was carried out, so that reviewers are not swayed by what they already know about the authors or institutions involved. Blinding may be successful in concealing identities and locations only some of the time. If an author is prominent in the field, his or her work can be easy to identify even without a name attached, and the same holds true for reviewers, whose identities may be disclosed by their style. In certain cases it is the circumstances of the study that make it possible to identify the authors. For example, if a cardiology study is carried out at a large, state-sponsored hospital in metropolitan Illinois, the researcher may be easy to track down, since there is only one such hospital in Illinois. Despite these limitations, blind review lets reviewers formulate objective evaluations of works under consideration.

Journals and university presses that are the first to see new research are in sensitive positions, especially with regard to potential conflicts of interest. For example, only a handful of researchers may be doing work in a particular area, and they often know one another and attend the same professional meetings. This does not mean that they always agree with one another—reviewers may be tempted to sabotage or hinder the work of rivals. Conflicts can be personal: researchers may not like one another. Conflicts can also be based on professional disagreements: researchers have profoundly different theoretical approaches to a problem. Editors try to rise above these disagreements and decide which articles ought to be published. Nevertheless, an unfavorable review can result in the article being returned to the author.

The review process allows scientists to see what competitors are doing with respect to new ideas and methodologies, and even bibliographic citations. Many journals try to contain this problem by requiring reviewers to treat documents under consideration for publication as privileged. That is, the reviewer makes no use of the information until it is available to others at publication. It is easy to see, though, how reviewers might be tempted to do otherwise.

Another problem that publishers face is duplicate publication, in which a researcher spreads findings out over a number of articles or presents data in a slightly different light several times. This does not necessarily consist of fraud or misrepresentation. It is simply that researchers divide their work to produce the maximum possible number of articles—a long list of published studies looks more impressive than a short list. The benefit of duplication is not to science but to the researcher whose primary goal is not contributing to knowledge but obtaining publicity, raises, and tenure. One defense of duplicate publication is that different journals have different audiences, and it is important to disseminate information widely through many publications. Increased ability of researchers to find published literature, however, no matter where it is published, makes duplicate publication harder and harder to defend.

Authorship

The nature of authorship in science can be problematic, although its problems have parallels elsewhere. Take novels or short stories as a model: the public may believe that an author writes the entire text on his or her own. But there are many "authors" behind any given text. Editors often make major revisions and changes to texts, even those of the most famous authors. In literary traditions, these editors usually are unnamed and their contributions are unpublicized. Some public figures hire ghostwriters, whose names never appear in the finished book. Payment for the service makes this arrangement acceptable to both parties. In contrast, authors of academic books often thank their editors and assistants in public acknowledgments. In almost all instances, a scientific text—and the efforts behind it—is the result of the work of many people.

With many involved in producing a scientific article, the ordering of authors' names becomes important. In scientific publications, tradition identifies two places in the list of names as especially noteworthy. The first place is one of greatest prominence, and the last place is by tradition a place of honor. The first author indicates the person whose work underlies the paper as a whole; the last name may indicate a person whose work or role made the study possible without necessarily doing the actual work. For example, the first author may be the graduate student who sets up the laboratory procedures, runs the study, collects and interprets the data, and writes the article. The last author may be the scientist in whose laboratory the student is working, whose grant supports the research, and whose suggestions guide the study to completion. Names between the two indicate people who have played one role or another, usually in descending order of importance. Disputes may obviously arise as to whose name should go where.

One standard is to list names according to the degree of contribution to the article, but even this is open to interpretation. For example, a senior scientist may conceive and direct a graduate student. The graduate student may do all the work, even to the point of drafting the article, but the senior scientist may wish to claim the position of lead author because it was after all his ideas that produced the study, and the study is part of his research program, including grant money, laboratory facilities, and constant stream of suggestions. The situation can go the other way too: it may be a graduate student whose ideas prove central to a study. Even so, the senior scientist may claim the position of lead author because, again, the study went forward in his laboratory.

Position in an author list is important for reasons unrelated to the article's content, namely, employment status, prestige, eligibility for research grants, and so on. These workers compete for places of honor, and vulnerable contributors, graduate students, for example, may be unrecognized with regard to the true extent of their contribution to a study. Thus they jockey to avoid the undistinguished middle of the list. It is increasingly common to see very long lists of names, reflecting all the people who may have had a hand in the design, conduct, and write-up of a study; however, some of these contributions may be minor if not completely trivial. Therefore, some journals require formal justification if the list of authors exceeds a certain number. Senior authors are encouraged to separate out substantial contributors from those who helped in minor ways. Some journals acknowledge the division of labor at the end of an article as follows:

Author Contributions

Study concept and design: Aileen Arlington, Brad Boylston

Acquisition of data: Christopher Copley

Analysis and interpretation of data: Darlene Dartmouth

Drafting of the manuscript: Eddie Exeter

Critical revision of the manuscript for important intellectual content: Frank Fairfield

Statistical expertise: Darlene Dartmouth

Obtained funding: Aileen Arlington

Administrative, technical, or material support: Larry Lansdowne

Study supervision: Bennie Beacon

This helps clarify the role of each named author and in many ways helps reduce tensions related to the order of names in the list.

It has sometimes happened that scientists use the names of others without their knowledge or consent. Adding the name of a prominent individual in the list of authors may increase its chance of being published. Most journals respond to this by requiring all named authors to affirm their participation in and responsibility for a study. This requirement may be extended even to people whose help is acknowledged in a note appended to the end of an article.

Embargoes

The timing of publication and use of published materials evokes ethical concern. Biomedical journals often ask that news media refrain from reporting findings until physicians have time to receive and review a study. They also ask authors to refrain from discussing results of their studies in public before the report is published. Journals do not want authors' promotion of their work in other venues to undercut the importance of the publication. Embargoes are seen as objectionable, however, when life-threatening conditions are at stake; if the information can be life saving, it should be made available as soon as possible. For this reason, journals and government health agencies issue "clinical alerts" if they determine that findings should be publicized before the official publication date.

That research results can and do have implications for clinical treatment has led some health activists to demand more immediate access to study results, even to receive preliminary reports as researchers file their data. It is clear, however, that the review process, with its time-consuming process of blind review, improves the quality and value of the reports before they are available to the scientific community and the public. It is likely that the need for time to evaluate and interest in access to data will remain in tension for the foreseeable future.

Use of Data Obtained in Unethical Ways

One ethical question that emerges after publication—sometimes well after—concerns data that were obtained in objectionable ways. One of the best-known debates in this area relates to data obtained by Nazi physicians and researchers who often subjected humans to agonizing interventions, even to the point of death, and certainly against their will. Many believe that the scientific community should not publish unethically obtained data, as this rewards the researchers by offering them outlets for their work. If unethically performed research is published, little incentive exists to avoid engaging in it. Another view is that such data may be used as a way of rescuing at least some shred of value from unethical experiments. In the case of some disputed work, it would be almost impossible to put the data back in the bottle. For example, it was alleged that studies distinguishing hepatitis A from hepatitis B were unethical because they were conducted with institutionally housed and disabled children at Willowbrook State School. Even if one agreed that those studies were unethical, it would be difficult to pretend that they had not had a positive result. Nevertheless, the debate about further use of unethically obtained data remains a live concern.

Many journals have formal policies that prohibit publication of such data, although limited use of the information may be allowed as long as it is accompanied by an advisory about the way in which it was obtained.[3] This accommodates both respect for human subjects who may have been abused while also putting the data to a use important to humanity. Data that are not ethically obtained are not always useful, but some of them are, and that utility keeps the debate alive.

References

1. David J. Miller, Michel Hersen, eds., *Research Fraud in the Behavioral and Biomedical Sciences* (New York: John Wiley, 1992).

2. Daniel J. Kevles, *The Baltimore Case: A Trial of Politics, Science, and Character* (New York: W.W. Norton, 1998).

3. Kristine Moe, "Should the Nazi Research Data Be Cited?" *Hastings Center Report*, Dec. 1984, pp. 5–7.

9.1

The Order of Authors' Names

The ordering of authors' names in scientific journals follows a convention not used elsewhere. The first author is usually the person who has done research essential to the study, and those that follow are ranked according to the importance of their contribution. The last name in the list is reserved as a place of honor for an essential contributor, for example, the researcher in whose laboratory the others worked, or who initiated the line of research. This author may have had very little to do with the actual study. As can be expected, contributors often jockey for position in the list.

Jose Delagarza was a postdoctoral fellow researching the way a particular disease progressed. He developed a hypothesis that a nontoxic substance might effectively treat certain aggressive forms of cancer while reducing the devastating side effects of conventional chemotherapy. To test his idea, he outlined a complex research plan. His postdoctoral advisor, Dr. Bill Cummings, supported this approach, but parts of Delagarza's proposal were beyond Cummings's expertise. Cummings, a nontenured assistant professor, suggested that Delagarza present his proposal during a department seminar to elicit suggestions from other faculty.

During the seminar, Dominick Cerino, PhD, head of the department in which both Cummings and Delagarza worked, showed great enthusiasm for the project, making several suggestions and encouraging Delagarza and Cummings to proceed.

Delagarza's pharmacological approach appeared to reduce the progression of tumors in animals. This study was almost certain to receive media attention when it appeared in the scientific journals. In the formal scientific report, Delagarza indicated Cummings as last author because Cummings had supervised the work on a day-to-day basis. He also knew this acknowledgment would help Cummings in his bid for tenure and promotion.

Cummings thought that it would be wise to show the manuscript to Cerino before submitting it to a prestigious journal, believing the department head would be proud of this breakthrough work. Moreover, Cerino was a member of the editorial board of the journal Delagarza hoped would publish the article. Although Cerino would not himself review the article, he might suggest reviewers who would be favorably disposed to the work. Cummings checked to ensure that Delagarza had acknowledged Cerino's helpful suggestions in the acknowledgment section of the paper, and asked Delagarza to show the paper to Cerino.

Cerino liked the manuscript but took notice of the acknowledgment of his suggestions. He insisted instead that he be listed as a coauthor, and, moreover, that his name appear last in the list (the senior author). He held that although he had not performed the experiments, his comments during seminars constituted the intellectual driving force behind Delagarza's work. Moreover, Cerino believed he had contributed by providing the scientific environment in which the study flourished. He had, after all, recruited Cummings to the department.

Dr. Cummings believed that he deserved senior author status because he had directly supervised Delagarza's work from beginning to end but was concerned that if he raised the issue, Cerino would retaliate by not supporting his promotion and tenure. Both Delagarza and Cummings knew that Dr. Cerino had an application to renew a grant pending before a federal funding agency. He would almost certainly report this new study in support of the application, primarily to signify his own value to the field. Dr. Cummings wondered if, when the day of publication came, Dr. Cerino would also want to hold a press conference to report the findings and if he, as senior author, would claim credit for the work.

Neither Delagarza nor Cummings was certain if they should let the matter drop or pursue it further. Delagarza, especially, did not want to raise a fuss, since hostility from Cerino could interfere with getting a job later on.

Study Questions

1. What are the nature and extent of Dr. Cerino's contribution to this article? Are they as extensive as he believes than to be?

2. Should Dr. Cerino be acknowledged as an author—in any sense—of this article?

3. Do you believe that the potential for retaliation is reason enough to accommodate Dr. Cerino's interest in being listed as senior author? If not, how might the postdoctoral fellow and junior faculty member respond to Cerino's claim to being senior author?

Prepared by Robert Folberg, Frances B. Geever Professor, Department of Pathology, University of Illinois College of Medicine at Chicago.

9.2

Authorship

In scientific publication, the tradition is that senior researchers are named last in the list of authors. This is especially true if junior faculty members or graduate students continue a line of work begun by that investigator. This custom raises concern, however, because the researcher's name is sometimes added even if he or she has not actively participated in the study. Other names may be added even for minor contributions. Some journals now require that the first author sign a statement taking responsibility for the entire article. They also ask for justification if more than five authors are listed. Most guidelines draw distinctions between first author, senior investigator, and so on. Standards for identifying contributors to research articles is evolving, and junior faculty and graduate students can be open to exploitation if they are not observed strictly.

1. To be listed as first author of an original scientific article, the investigator must (a) have adapted a general hypothesis (his or her own or the senior author's) in a detailed, systematic fashion, down to the actual details of Methods and Materials; (b) have participated in a major way in the analysis and interpretation of data; and (c) have written the paper. It is desirable, but not obligatory, that the first author also participated substantially in performing research and data collection.

2. To be listed as a coauthor, an investigator must be recognized as having made significant contributions to the planning and execution of the research, methods and procedures, collection and analysis of data, and so forth.

3. To be listed last as a senior author, a scientist must (a) have either formulated the original general hypotheses or provided significant intellectual resources for the work, (b) have provided constructive criticism of the paper during and/or after its composition, (c) accept overall responsibility for all the findings of the final version of the paper and for the order of authorship, and (d) have provided the laboratory space and/or finances for the experiment.

Study Questions

1. A prominent botanist directs several of his senior graduate students to review some data he has collected over the past two years and draft an article describing it. Three students do this work: one compiles tables and another describes the significance of the work. The third student, who finds writing very easy, writes a twenty-page draft of an article. The botanist spends an hour and a half reviewing the article and makes a few additions and corrections. He tells yet another graduate student to write an abstract and send it out for publication. According to the guidelines above, how should the botanist be listed as author?

2. Sally Smith is eager to please her biochemistry mentor who is notorious for sloppy habits. He asks her to piece together an article from some notes he gave her. Drawing up the draft required her to do some background research, confirm the accuracy of all citations, and, when reviewing lab notes, correct mistaken entries. All told, she spends about seven days putting

the article into final form. Her mentor thanks her profusely for her efforts; however, when he sends the article out for publication, he does not list her as a coauthor. He does acknowledge her for identifying useful materials. According to the guidelines above, is Sally Smith entitled to be listed as an author?

From *University of Virginia Guidelines for Authorship*, reprinted in R. Scott Jones, John C. Fletcher, "Self-Regulation of Surgical Practice and Research," in Laurence B. McCullough, James W. Jones, Baruch A. Brody, eds., *Surgical Ethics* (New York: Oxford University Press, 1998), pp. 255–279.

9.3

Reporting Scientific Advances

One of the most popular armchair sports among researchers is bashing the media. Researchers criticize the media for hasty, inaccurate, and oversimplified coverage. The passage below faults journalists for their easy acceptance of scientific reports. It charges that journalism has abdicated its responsibilities to do aggressive investigation in science reporting. If this criticism is accurate, it suggests the public is profoundly compromised in its understanding of scientific advances.

"Science writers in effect are brokers, framing social reality for their readers and shaping the public consciousness about science-related events. Through their selection of news about science and technology they set the agenda for public policy. Through their presentation of science news they lay the foundation for personal attitudes and public actions. For they are often our only source of information about the technical choices that significantly affect our lives . . .

"Too often science is presented as an arcane activity outside and above the sphere of normal human understanding, and therefore beyond our control. Too often the coverage is promotional and uncritical, encouraging apathy, a sense of impotence and the ubiquitous tendency to defer to expertise. . . . There is little in this type of reporting to help the reader understand the nature of scientific evidence and the difference between science and unverified opinion. As a result, when new problems emerge as the focus of public concern, people are ill prepared to deal with scientific information. The persistent fear of catching AIDS through casual contact with AIDS victims despite scientific evidence to the contrary is a case in point . . .

"Some science writers are in awe of scientists; others are intimidated. But most are bewildered by the complexity of technical issues. The difficulty of evaluating a complex and uncertain subject converges with the day-to-day constraints of the journalistic profession to reinforce the tendency to rely uncritically on scientific expertise . . . Thus while art, theater, music, and literature are routinely subjected to criticism, science and technology are almost always spared . . . Unaggressive in their reporting and relying on official sources, science journalists present a narrow range of coverage. Many journalists are, in effect, retailing science and technology more than investigating them, identifying with their sources more than challenging them."

Study Questions

1. How convincing is the argument that science reporting is not sufficiently critical? Can you think of any instances in which reporters should have been more aggressive in challenging scientists' reports or research initiatives?

2. What might journalism do to promote more critical evaluation of the nature and value of research? Is it the case that an impassable gap must exist between the public and researchers?

3. To what extent do you think it is true that much science journalism is cheerleading for researchers? If journalism usually fails to be sufficiently critical of research, what alternatives are there for achieving critical oversight of what scientists are doing?

Quoted with minor changes from Dorothy Nelkin, "The High Cost of Hype," in Ruth Ellen Bulger, Elizabeth Heitman, Stanley Joel Reiser, eds., *The Ethical Dimensions of the Biological Sciences* (Cambridge: Cambridge University Press, 1993), pp. 270–277.

9.4

Origins of Fraud

Every so often a scandal involving fraudulent biomedical data occupies the news media. The commentary below offers a theory about why fraud occurs in the clinical sciences. Whether this account is complete, and whether the suggested remedies will prevent fraud, are key issues for discussion.

The origins of fraud in medical studies can be traced to three main causes. The first is hypercompetitiveness in medical school for grades and honors. Studies show that even in medical school, students cheat in various ways, not only on exams but also in aspects of patient care.

The second main source is the size of the scientific enterprise itself. There is so much science that it is impossible to provide the kind of oversight that is necessary to squelch the temptation to report false data. In particular, inexperienced junior researchers are often left to their own devices because senior researchers and administrators do not have time to review every research project.

A third source of fraud lies in competition for grants and academic rewards. Grants are essential to promotion, and they are fiercely pursued. But academic promotion only makes things worse, because researchers are always mindful of what new grants and publications will do to help their careers, especially when it comes to tenure.

None of these sources means that fraud is inevitable. On the contrary, it may be preventable if principal investigators take on more responsibility to ensure that their associates are committed to the truth, and if data are checked at several levels by competent people. Fraud is all the more reprehensible in scientists who by their career choice have committed themselves to the discovery and dissemination of truth. At the institutional level, mechanisms must be in place to sort out fraud, and administrators should be sufficiently familiar with laboratories under their direction to know how to investigate should a question of fraud arise.

Study Questions

1. How convincing are these primary reasons why people commit fraud in clinical research?

2. If competition prompts fraud, what steps might be taken to reduce it for medical students? For example, perhaps medical schools could identify and admit students who are most cooperative rather than the most competitive. What else might be done in this regard?

3. Science is considered to be a self-correcting effort. That is, it will eventually uncover fraud because its methods require independent confirmation of research reports. How accurate is this characterization, and does it mean that fraud committed in clinical research is not especially worrisome?

Adapted from Robert G. Petersdorf, "The Pathogenesis of Fraud in Medical Science," *Annals of Internal Medicine* 1986 (104): 252–254.

Repetitive Publication

It is universally agreed that academic researchers are under enormous pressure to publish. Publication is the pathway to tenure, promotion, professional prestige, and financial reward. In a sense, scientists should be pressured to publish, because publication makes it possible to evaluate scientific claims. For publicly funded research, publication serves as a return on that investment. That said, publication is not merely a way of communicating with like-minded researchers. Some researchers try to extend their publications because of its many rewards. This incentive creates several problems.

"*Repetitive publication*—republishing essentially the same content in successive papers or in chapters, reviews, and other papers—also wastes resources. In one episode involving this journal about two years ago, we published a paper about a serious adverse pulmonary effect due to a new cardiovascular drug. A paper published in a radiological journal five months later described the same effect in apparently the same patients.

"The authors of the two papers were different, but the papers came from the same medical school. Case details strongly suggested that the same cases had been reported twice. At least one author of the second paper must have been aware of the first paper because that author had been acknowledged for reviewing it. An excuse for this duplication might have been to get the message to two audiences unlikely to see each other's journals. But is the cost of duplicating the message for two audiences justified?

"For some decades the cost of searching through secondary services for information in a journal not usually seen by the searcher might have justified such duplicative publication. Now, the ease, speed, and relatively low cost of searching scientific literature through online bibliographic services discredit this excuse. One good reason to object to the repetition in this episode is that the re-reporting of the four cases misrepresents the incidence of adverse drug effects. A literature search would turn up eight cases instead of four. A closely related abuse is producing the papers I call 'meat extenders,' papers that add data to the author's previously reported data, without reaching new conclusions.

"None of these abuses is dramatically unethical in the sense that fakery and fraud are. The scientific community might not even agree on whether repetitive and duplicative publication are unethical. Wasteful publication might be seen as justified by needs to compete for institutional and financial support to ensure academic survival."

Study Questions

1. Why is it an ethical problem to engage in repetitive publication? How serious are the alleged consequences of repetitive publication?
2. How convincing is it that repetitive publication is not only harmless but is necessary in order to reach different audiences?

Quoted from Edward J. Huth, "Irresponsible Authorship and Wasteful Publication," *Annals of Internal Medicine* 1986 (104): 257–259.

9.6

When Industry Does Not Like Published Findings

The case below raises questions about publication standards when an article evokes not merely criticism but also threats of legal action against wrongful conduct. A journal formally retracted an article, although apparently without the knowledge or consent of the authors.

In fall of 1998, the University of Denver's *Denver Journal of International Law and Policy* published an article by William A. Wines, Mark A. Buchanan, and Donald J. Smith. The article called for legal reform in light of certain practices of transnational corporations, and cited Boise Cascade Corporation in particular.

In response to letters from Boise Cascade, administration officials at the University of Denver retracted the article in 1999, asking two major online legal databases to remove it. In its summer 1999 issue, the journal published a notice that the article had been retracted because of lack of scholarship and false content.

In March 2000, Boise Cascade notified the authors of these events and demanded that the authors "immediately cease distributing copies of the article and immediately stop making false and defamatory statements about Boise Cascade." Following protests from the authors, University of Denver officials said they had no choice but to retract the article after determining it had been a serious mistake to publish it.

The article alleged that Boise Cascade was typical of transnational companies in greed and arrogance. It cited irresponsibility and indifference to the consequences of shutting down a large lumber mill in Idaho and opening a much cheaper operation in Mexico. It further concluded that the company ignored unsafe working conditions in that Mexico mill. The authors also disputed the propriety of locating the Mexico mill in an area already embroiled in timber disputes. Boise Cascade believed the article implicated the company in the death of people killed in those disputes.

The University of Denver claimed that the article did not meet editorial standards and was in fact not well suited for the journal. A lawyer for the university acknowledged that Boise Cascade's objections did meet the standard for bringing a lawsuit, and it appeared that the company was prepared to sue. Other university officials insisted that the decision to retract the article was made independently and in response to threats of lawsuits. The authors said that they have yet to receive a formal identification of problems that led to the retraction. A spokesperson for Human Rights Watch objected to the retraction as well: "Within the bounds of truth and good form, there's no reason for law journals not to be forums for strong social commentary. One should be able to criticize people who are doing not very nice things."

Study Questions

1. Do you think that the editors and sponsors of a professional journal should retract an article without putting allegations of error before the authors?

2. From statements made by officials after the publication, do you believe that the journal adequately reviewed the content of the article? What editorial standards might have been overlooked in publishing this article?

3. Should the journal have offered the authors the opportunity to reply to its actions and to the allegations by Boise Cascade?

Adapted from Peter Monaghan, "A Journal Article Is Expunged and Its Authors Cry Foul," *Chronicle of Higher Education,* Dec. 8, 2000, pp. A14–A16, A18.

9.7

Embargoes of Scientific Reports

At many scientific journals, it is standard policy to put embargoes on what authors can say about their work before publication. This is done for a variety of reasons; for example, to protect the public by ensuring that research goes through a peer-review process. However, embargoes also protect the economic interests of the journal since they limit availability of the information, and thus the journal becomes the authoritative source. Embargoes also help promote the newsworthiness of scientific reports.

Journals usually treat the manuscripts they receive as confidential while deciding whether or not to publish them. They also insist that this material be kept confidential among authors, editorial staff, and anonymous reviewers. Journals ask authors to refrain from informing others (colleagues, professional organizations, news media) that their articles are under consideration or have been accepted and are awaiting publication. To publish scientific results, journals require that the material not have been published elsewhere, including not only other scientific journals, but news coverage and postings on the Internet. However, there are exceptions to these principles of confidentiality and no previous publication.

For example, authors are entitled to make preliminary reports at scientific meetings, but they may be urged not to circulate complete drafts of their work. They are asked to limit conversations with the media, if science reporters are present, to material they have presented formally. Publication of short abstracts of the work in conference proceedings is acceptable, but authors are often directed not to hold press conferences about their work or to issue press releases.

Authors are entitled to present their work before government agencies such as the FDA. They are also entitled to post notices of adverse reactions of drugs to relevant government agencies without violating the rule of no prior publication. If researchers identify information that is of keen importance to the public health, journals may permit publicity about that information and not jeopardize publication, as long as the researchers work with the journal and relevant government agencies. Some journals have means to expedite the review process and to publish findings on Web sites rather than wait for print publication.

Journals may employ embargoes; that is, agreements that the news media not report on articles until a certain time. For example, the *Journal of the American Medical Association* asks that news media not publicize material in its weekly issue until 3 P.M. on the day before the formal publication. A week before that time, however, the journal may send copies to physicians and the news media. According to the journal, "The embargo policy is intended to enable physicians to have access to the published articles several days before news coverage occurs so they will be prepared if patients ask them about news reports based on a published article." The embargo also gives reporters time to prepare stories. Researchers can cooperate with journalists as they prepare their stories, but they should do so only on the understanding that the reporters will abide by the embargo. Ordinarily, journals stipulate that dissemination of new medical information should coincide with formal publication dates.

Study Questions

1. In an age of Internet communication, do embargoes work against scientific openness and the dissemination of important health information? Do they slow transmission of information to people who need it, perhaps even jeopardizing their health? What is the merit of embargoes against disclosure and discussion of scientific reports before their formal publication?

2. A former editor of the *Journal of the American Medical Association* commented that its policy sounded "heavy-handed" and worried that it could "intimidate" younger researchers. Others noted that in the 1980s the journal published commentary that criticized embargoes just like the one they were adopting. Some critics argued that the benefit of embargoes falls on journals that can then maintain their prestige and increase revenue through subscriptions. How serious are these criticisms? Are they serious enough to scrap existing embargo policies and find an alternative?

See P. B. Fontanarosa, A. Flanagin, C. D. DeAngelis, "The *Journal*'s Policy Regarding Release of Information to the Public," *Journal of the American Medical Association* 2000 (284): 2929–2931. See also Lawrence K. Altman, "Medical Journal Bars Authors' Prepublication Comments," *New York Times,* Dec. 13, 2000.

9.8

Medical Advertising

Pharmaceutical companies carry out ambitious advertising campaigns. Some are directed toward consumers, others toward physicians who prescribe drugs. Biomedical journals are a prime means to reach physicians through such advertising. The commentary below questions lack of oversight that journals give to information in pharmaceutical advertising. The ethical question is whether the advertising revenue received by a medical journal sways the judgment of the journal or physicians in a way that might distort research findings.

Medical journals closely scrutinize the contents of their articles. They do not, however, exert the same scrutiny with regard to advertising that supports them. Most journals admit that it would be difficult to stay solvent without support of advertisements. That said, advertisements contain many assertions that journals do not check for accuracy.

Some editors say that they not only lack the resources to check advertisements for accuracy but that doing so would put the journals in the position of appearing to endorse some products, which they do not want to do. These editors maintain that federal regulations regarding medical advertising are—and should be—the front line of defense against deceptive advertising.

Study Questions

1. Are you convinced that medical journals should take steps to ensure the accuracy of all statements contained in advertisements in their pages?

2. How convincing is the belief that checking facts would be seen, rightly or wrongly, as lending endorsement to the medical drugs and devices being advertised?

3. It is worth wondering whether revenue from advertisers influences the content of journals. Is it likely that subtle pressure from advertisers might influence journals to print data favorable to sponsors' products or to suppress unfavorable data?

Adapted from David S. Shimm, Roy G. Spece, Jr., Michelle Burpeau DiGregorio, "Conflicts of Interests in Relationships between Physicians and the Pharmaceutical Industry," in Roy G. Spece, David S. Schimm, Allen E. Buchanan, eds., *Conflicts of Interest in Clinical Practice and Research* (New York: Oxford University Press, 1996), pp. 321–357.

When a Subject Recognizes Himself in a Scientific Report

What should happen to researchers who do not observe standards of informed consent or who fail to protect subject confidentiality in scientific reports? A subject was greatly upset to recognize himself in a case report published by a prominent psychologist. Not only had he not given permission for his case to be published, he believed that he could be identified from the article. In highly specific case studies, subjects might in fact be able to recognize themselves.

Charlie Gordon (a pseudonym) was born in 1947 with congenital hypothyroidism, a condition that leads to stunted physical growth and mental retardation. At age two years, he received an experimental therapy of cow hormone replacement that led to considerable physical and mental development.

At the psychohormonal research center at Johns Hopkins University in Baltimore, psychologist John Money began to follow Charlie Gordon's development starting when the boy was five and continuing for the next twenty-five years. During that time, Charlie's I.Q. moved from 84 at age five to 127. Gordon believed that Money's involvement was intended to help him cope with difficulties associated with his hypothyroidism.

In 1989 Gordon ran across a book by Money, *Vandalized Lovemaps,* in which he recognized himself as the subject of a section called "Pedophilia in a Male with a History of Hypothyroidism." Over the years Money had conducted interviews with Gordon about his sexual interests and behaviors. Gordon had talked about masturbation techniques, his involvement in three-way sexual affairs, and his interest in girls much younger than himself. He even confessed that because of insecurities about his small stature, he sought relationships with younger partners, once with a fourteen-year-old girl.

Gordon was shocked to see extensive quotations from therapy sessions as well as a diagnosis of pedophilia applied to him. The book also quoted his father as saying his mother had sex with her brother. Although he was not specifically named, Gordon was sure anyone who knew him or his family would recognize them.

Gordon tried to complain to Money to no avail. He then complained to the National Institutes of Health, whose Office for Protection from Research Risks found that Money had never secured consent for Gordon's involvement as a research subject. The office also agreed that persons acquainted with him could have identified Gordon from the text. They directed Johns Hopkins University to republish guidelines for safeguarding the identity of research subjects. They also directed that Money apologize to Gordon in the presence of his department chair. Gordon says he never got that apology.

Study Questions

1. How serious are the effects of Charlie Gordon discovering his case history in a book? How might his interests be compromised?

2. It can be agreed that Gordon should have been asked about his willingness to be treated as a research subject. Nevertheless, it remains true that cases in all their detail are interesting and important to researchers. Is it necessarily a bad thing that subjects may recognize themselves in published case studies?

3. After the finding of ethical lapses, do you believe that a stronger response should be required from Money other than a verbal apology that may or may not have happened?

Adapted from John Colapinto, *As Nature Made Him: The Boy Who Was Raised as a Girl* (New York: HarperCollins, 2000), pp. 240–244.

Graduate Students as Authors

In the hypothetical case below, the veracity of quotations used in a study of lynching comes into question. It is unclear, however, that a mechanism exists by which this question could be brought to resolution, since graduate students often have little control over the use of their work and do not have the independence and protection that come with professorship.

Professor Ashley Jefferson studies U.S. Southern culture and is at work on a study of race and lynching. By all accounts, this study will receive wide attention when it is finished. Jefferson relies on graduate students to examine archives and to conduct some interviews. One of those graduate students, Patrick Rowe, conducted three in-person interviews with Sadie Jones, an elderly African-American woman who witnessed several lynchings in her youth, including the killing of her cousin.

Through a friend, Rowe learns that Jefferson gave a presentation about these interviews during an academic conference on race and quoted Jones's poetic statements about brotherhood and redemption. Rowe said this was odd, because in the interviews he handed over to Jefferson, Jones had done little more than quote Scripture and talk about God's will. In fact, he doesn't remember that Jones said anything worth while at all. Where had these memorable statements come from? He was at a loss to say, because Jefferson never sent him a copy of the presentation.

The friend suggests that Rowe look into the matter because Jefferson mentioned him as a coauthor. Because Rowe discusses the matter with a number of friends in his department, word about his concern filters back to Jefferson. Jefferson recommends to the department head that Rowe not be rehired, saying his interviews were shallow. What's more, Jefferson says he himself had to reinterview Jones to have her open up and share her sharp insight and clear recollections of the lynchings. The department head raises no concern here, but he does remind Jefferson that the student should be listed as a coauthor on any publications to which he contributed. Jefferson assures him he has already seen to this.

The department head then asks whether Jefferson's tape recordings of interviews with Jones could be made available for an online presentation of the department's works. The department head says it would be scintillating to hear that woman talk about the lynchings in her own voice and with her own charged language. Jefferson regrets he can't help the department, because his tape recorder wasn't working when he telephoned Jones. He has only some of the notes he took immediately after their conversation.

Study Questions

1. As a graduate student and employee, Patrick Rowe faces certain hurdles in trying to clarify the origin of interviews ascribed to Sadie Jones. What actions should he take if he believes that the content of the interviews has been falsified?

2. Professor Jefferson is not under obligation to record every interview on audiotape. Because he has not recorded his calls to Jones, do you believe that misconduct or evidence of retaliation could be meaningfully ascertained if an investigation were to be launched?

Originally prepared by Vicki Field, Peggy Sundermeyer, Ken Pimple, Indiana University. Adapted by Timothy F. Murphy. A longer version of this case may be found at http://php. indiana.edu/~pimple/. Follow the link to "Adventures in Collaborative Research."

A Question of Theft?

It is an ideal in the scientific community that sharing work is essential to progress. That ideal has come under fire for a variety of reasons, not the least of which is that scientific work has economic implications that may not have been so pronounced in the past. Scientific results are used for career advancement, prestige, and monetary gain, and these rewards cut into the willingness of researchers to share materials openly.

Before the advent of new methods of molecular biology, Professor Yousef Darwish had studied several disorders with morphological techniques that were available. He hypothesized that several conditions that were considered to be separate disorders might, in fact, be related to one another in terms of their etiology (causal origin). His laboratory continued to work in this area, and in the 1990s, he began to employ molecular tools that could permit him to validate his hypothesis. He planned to submit a proposal to a federal funding agency within eighteen months.

Professor Joyce Porter was a researcher at a nearby university, and she knew Darwish from conferences they attended together. They were friendly but did not know one another well. At one point, Porter asked Darwish if she could use some of his electron micrographs for a seminar that she would be giving to her graduate students. Darwish was flattered that his work was attracting attention from a colleague, and he provided Porter with the material she requested.

Approximately one year later Darwish learned that Porter received a substantial grant from a federal agency to study the hypothesis that he had been investigating for a decade. He also learned from a graduate student who saw a presentation by Porter that she used his photomicrographs in her application for the grant. Darwish made a few phone calls to friends at Porter's university, and from what he could piece together, Porter made no mention of Darwish as the source of the photographs. And she certainly did not tell him she intended to use the materials this way. Darwish was concerned that his ability to secure funding for his own research might be jeopardized because the scientific community now looked to Porter as the preeminent authority in the field, and because his own application for funding would essentially duplicate Porter's and would not be considered new.

Study Questions

1. Is Professor Porter guilty of wrongful use of Professor Darwish's materials, and if so, how serious is this misuse?

2. What actions should Darwish take in response to his belief that his work was stolen?

3. If it turns out that Porter did use Darwish's materials to prepare her grant application, do you believe that is enough reason for a funding agency to turn that application down?

9.12

Responsibility for Data

Senior researchers often rely on the work of many persons in their laboratories to help them prepare, conduct, and interpret the results of experiments. They are almost never in a position to oversee each detail of the studies closely, although they are responsible for the studies as a whole. The case below involves discrepancies that one assistant discovered in the work of another.

Jack Eklov, PhD, hired Ms. Fadden, a master's degree student, to help with animal studies in his laboratory. As usual, Dr. Eklov was particularly busy with a number of projects. He had closely supervised Ms. Fadden and had always found her records to be meticulous and accurate. When Ms. Fadden wanted to return to England to complete work toward her master's degree, Dr. Eklov immediately recruited a replacement for her.

Several months later, Dr. Eklov submitted a manuscript based on experiments in which Ms. Fadden played a role. While the paper was undergoing peer review, Ms. Fadden's replacement, Adam Krafsur, noticed some discrepancies in Ms. Fadden's log books and called this to the attention of Dr. Eklov. The discrepancies were minor and most likely originated from unintentional error rather than a deliberate attempt to alter data. Eklov traced the dates of the experiments, however, and discovered that the manuscript under review was based in part on these erroneous findings.

Eklov found himself in a difficult situation. He was fairly certain that the discrepancies were minor, but he could not be entirely certain that they did not influence data analyses that were so important to the manuscript. He attempted to contact Ms. Fadden but she had married and was away from her laboratory for an extended period of time. It was impossible for him to repeat all of the experiments in which Ms. Fadden played a role to verify that the statements made in the paper were correct.

Eklov was not sure if he should recall the paper from editorial review, as he was not sure that the discrepancies were serious.

Study Questions

1. What is the rationale for Eklov writing to the journal immediately and advising the editors of his doubts, telling them that he will contact them later if it turns out the discrepancies are, in fact, serious?

2. Should Eklov wait to talk to Ms. Fadden before making a decision about what to do next, including withdrawing the paper? What advantages and disadvantages would that approach have?

Prepared by Robert Folberg, Frances B. Geever Professor, Department of Pathology, University of Illinois College of Medicine at Chicago.

From Class Report to Formal Study

Research often begins in ways that do not require review and approval by IRBs. Many projects undertaken for classroom purposes—interviews, for example—may lead to results that investigators realize might be useful for publication. The following study began as a classroom project and was turned into formal publication. It used existing data taken from confidential interviews.

Some men have sex in public places (restrooms, parking lots, clubs, etc.), and it was suggested that they do so because of social oppression. According to this theory if society were not hostile toward homosexuality, men would have opportunities to socialize with one another in other ways and have sex in more discreet locations. Some locations in the United States show little social hostility toward homosexuality, yet men continue to use public venues to have sex with other men. One college student wanted to know why and to test the theory that social oppression is a contributing cause.

In 1998 and 1999, for a class project, the student interviewed ten men who had at some point used "glory holes" for sex. Glory hole is a slang term for a hole in the partition of a wall, through which men have oral and sometimes anal sex. These glory holes can be found in public restrooms and in sex clubs. The student wanted to know what these men found attractive about this kind of sexual experience.

The student recruited subjects through his friends and knew them to be self-identified gay men. He told them their "explicit testimony" would be used but not rewarded or credited in any way. Their identities would remain confidential. In one instance, he began his interview in the presence of another man who agreed to be interviewed as well. Later, the student decided to turn the class project into a formal journal article. When publishing the study, he identified his subjects in a very broad way: "a forty-year-old European man," "an American man in his fifties," "a man in his late twenties," and so on. He made no mention of whether these interviews were recorded or what the disposition of interview materials might have been. Nor did he state whether or not the subjects were identified more explicitly in his notebooks.

The researcher did not use a structured interview, but asked a variety of open-ended questions ("Have you used glory holes? " "Where and how?"). Some subjects were hesitant to describe their experiences directly. Nevertheless, no one withdrew as the student asked the men if they found using glory holes exciting because it was dangerous, the kinds of sexual activities they performed, the genitalia they found especially attractive, and the overall importance of glory holes to their sexual lives. The student concluded that the men had a variety of reasons for using glory holes, not many of which were connected to social oppression.

Study Questions

1. It was not the student's original intention to publish a formal report of his findings. If he had intended to publish his findings from the beginning, what differences in procedure would you recommend he take to ensure informed consent and confidentiality?

2. Information collected for one purpose is often useful for another purpose. What exactly did these subjects originally consent to? Should the student have gone back to the subjects and asked for consent to use their interviews as part of a published study?

3. Journals face questions of whether to publish reports that rely on data that was not collected in ways that would satisfy ethics committees. Given the way data were collected in this study, would you recommend that a journal accept this article for publication?

Adapted from Don Bapst, "Glory Holes and the Men Who Use Them," *Journal of Homosexuality* 2001 (41): 89–102.

Matching Punishment to Misconduct

The case below describes a scientist who misrepresented his publications when applying for a grant from the federal government. Whereas a good deal of thought has been expended on how to identify and deter misconduct, less attention is paid to how to sanction researchers found to have falsified documents.

In 2000, the Office of Research Integrity at the National Institutes of Health (NIH) found that Michael K. Hartzer, an associate professor of biomedical sciences at Oakland University in Rochester, Michigan, had made a series of misstatements about his published academic record. In the course of applying for eight NIH grants, Professor Hartzer listed eleven article manuscripts as either accepted for publication or in press. The term "accepted" means that a journal has agreed to publish the article but has not specified a time for publication. "In press" indicates that a manuscript has been accepted and is being edited and otherwise prepared for imminent publication. Investigators at both Oakland University and the Office for Research Integrity found that these eleven articles had in fact been rejected at the time of the grant application or were never published.

Hartzer accepted these findings and entered into a Voluntary Exclusion Agreement with the Public Health Service (PHS), the administrative oversight department of NIH. This means that for a period of three years, beginning on November 20, 2000, he cannot serve in any advisory capacity to PHS. He cannot serve on review committees, as a consultant, or in any other capacity. Furthermore, in future grant applications, both Hartzer and his employing institution must *certify* that all manuscripts and publications are properly and accurately represented.

Study Questions

1. When Michael Hartzer falsified his academic publications when applying for federal grant support, what actions were taken against him?

2. Do you believe that these actions were appropriate? Why or why not?

3. Do you believe that such sanction is sufficiently strong to dissuade others from falsifying their applications for grant support?

Adapted from an on-line report issued by the National Institutes of Health (www.nih.gov) on December 12, 2000. The NIH routinely reports misconduct findings on its Web pages.

9.15

Use of Nazi Data: Pernkopf's *Atlas*

What use, if any, may be made of scientific materials produced in an unethical manner? Several instances from World War II raise this question in very pointed ways. The case below raises this question with regard to a work with durable value: a medical atlas that shows various tissues, organs, and systems and is widely recognized as a significant accomplishment in its own right.

Beginning in the 1930s, Eduard Pernkopf began to produce *The Atlas of Topographic and Applied Human Anatomy,* an extensive study of human anatomy. This multivolume atlas featured anatomical drawings made by several artists. It was highly regarded for the quality of its artistic accomplishment and educational value. It has been translated into a variety of languages and is still in use.

There is no doubt that Pernkopf was an ardent Nazi, and in the 1990s his atlas came under fire. A United States physician argued that many people would have been killed and their bodies used in the preparation of drawings and paintings of body parts. Clear evidence from the period showed that researchers had little difficulty obtaining human subjects from concentration camps for all manner of "experiments" and purposes. However, evidence that Pernkopf obtained bodies this way was circumstantial. It may be that no definitive method is available to trace the source of the bodies used for the atlas.

In response to the protest, some medical libraries withdrew this book from circulation, at least for a time. Others did not and kept it on their shelves. The publisher said that a commemoration of the dead should be observed as it became established who they were and how they were victimized. Others pointed out that other German anatomists were Nazis as well, and that if consistency was the issue, no atlases from this era should be used. One even proposed that the book should be used as a way of conferring dignity on the subjects who may have been killed as part of its production: "The atlas very much belongs in our daily lives, that we may not become complacent, much less forgetful."

Study Questions

1. Although the physician asking for the withdrawal of Pernkopf's atlas had no direct evidence that people were killed to produce these volumes, do you believe that it is reasonable to believe that this probably did happen?

2. What is the best reason not to use Pernkopf's atlas?

3. Do you believe that using the anatomy atlas for educational and other purposes would confer some measure of dignity on those who might have been killed for its production?

Adapted from Garrett Riggs, "What Should We Do with Pernkopf's Atlas?" *Academic Medicine* 1998 (September): 380–386. See also Nicholas Wade, "Doctors Question Use of Nazi Medical Atlas," *New York Times,* Nov. 26, 1996, B7; and R. S. Panush, "Letter," *Journal of the American Medical Association* 1996 (276): 1633.

Use of Nazi Data: Hypothermia Studies

Nazi researchers felt little compunction about exposing prisoners to grotesque and inhuman suffering. The lead United States prosecutor at the Nuremberg trials, Telford Taylor, said, "These experiments revealed nothing that civilized medicine can use." That was something of an overstatement because some of the data could be used at least in indirect ways. For example, researchers could use data from hypothermia studies to estimate the likelihood of survival after people were capsized into frigid ocean waters. One legacy of these experiments is the debate about whether and to what extent research data should be used when gained under immoral circumstances.

Robert Pozos was director of the Hypothermia Laboratory at the University of Minnesota in Duluth, and in that capacity studied methods of resuscitating people who had been subjected to very low temperatures. For the most part, information about rewarming techniques has been gathered in a nonsystematic way. Controversy surrounds the best way to rewarm people who suffer from extreme hypothermia. Various techniques are used, and it is not certain whether physicians should rely primarily on the person's own body heat (passive rewarming) or on application of heat from other sources (active rewarming). Relatively little published research in this area is available to help determine which procedures to follow. Pozos did conduct experiments on human subjects in his laboratory, but he did not allow a subject's temperature to drop more than 36°, as that would be highly dangerous.

Some Nazi researchers had, however, done exactly that and attempted various rewarming techniques. One worked on developing "rapid active rewarming" involving hot liquids. These experiments involved immersing naked prisoners in tanks of ice water. In fact, many subjects died.

Dr. Pozos gathered and analyzed the data from these experiments that he knew could not be conducted ethically at the present time. In fact, he wanted to publish this information. He was well aware of the circumstances under which the data were obtained. In justifying publication, he said, "It could advance my work in that it takes human subjects farther than we're willing."

Study Questions

1. Some maintain that medical journals should not publish unethically obtained data. In fact, however, citations of the Nazi hypothermia studies are not rare. Do you think it is important to exclude these data from publication?

2. Kristine Moe has said that the data produced by unethical Nazi experiments may be used only when the scientific validity of the data is clear and only if there is no alternative source of the same data. Do you think this is an acceptable viewpoint?

3. Robert J. Levine has held that it is acceptable to publish Nazi data and other suspect data if they are used in a scientifically meaningful way. When publishing the material, journals should, however, also publish an editorial identifying the ways in which the data are ethically

problematic. The journals should also invite a response to the editorial from the author(s) of the article. All three items—study, editorial, and response to the editorial—should be published simultaneously. Do you think this is a reasonable approach to resolving problems associated with unethically obtained data, or does it still create a market for unethical studies?

Adapted from Kristine Moe, "Should the Nazi Research Data Be Cited?" *Hastings Center Report*, Dec. 1984, pp. 5–7. See also Barry Siegel, "Can Evil Beget Good? Nazi Data: A Dilemma for Science," *Los Angeles Times*, Oct. 30, 1988.

Graduate School Blues

What should happen to researchers who fail to comply with oversight standards? The case below raises the instance of an eager graduate student who got ahead of the process, possibly as a result of poor institutional advisement, and put his degree in jeopardy as a result.

Thom Jessell works as a nursing instructor at a small community college and is pursuing a master's degree in sociology at an on-line university. He has never set foot on the campus of the university that will award him his degree. To complete the requirements for his project, Jessell is studying the impact of educational videos on the perceptions of race among nursing students at the hospital. He devises a questionnaire that students will fill out before and after watching a video. The students will sign their name to the questionnaire, but Jessell intends to use the names only to link the prevideo and postvideo results. It is of no interest to him how individual subjects did or did not change their views because of the video. His goal is to see whether the short video made students more comfortable about dealing with patients of various races. He receives approval from the director of nursing studies to show the video and conduct the surveys in a regularly scheduled nursing classes.

After his project was done, Jessell learned that his university required review and approval of all studies. He did not realize that he had to receive approval before beginning something so harmless as this educational study. His advisor made no mention of this requirement. Jessell had no interest in publishing anything; he only wanted to use the data for his master's degree. To meet the requirement, he therefore filed for approval of the research. The IRB advised him that they could not grant approval after the fact. They also stated that if Jessell wanted to publish the findings, he should disclose to any journals that he conducted the research without IRB approval. This was discouraging because the video was extremely helpful to nursing students, and this result should be known to nursing educators. He wondered whether he could bypass the IRB by simply writing a letter to the editor of a nursing journal and telling them the ways in which he found the video useful. He believed this would not be the same as submitting a formal study.

Jessell was worried, furthermore, that he might not be permitted to obtain his master's degree because he violated policy. He could not find anything on-line about the university's policies in such a situation. He wondered whether he should ask his advisor whether or not his degree was in jeopardy. But he also wondered whether he would be better off if he had just stayed quiet and not raised a red flag. After all, the IRB had said nothing to him about his degree.

Study Questions

1. Do you believe that work carried out for a class project or a master's thesis should undergo review from an ethics committee?

2. In what way might the results of this study be sensitive, and did the researcher do enough to protect the confidentiality of his subjects?

3. Are you convinced that this student should be denied a master's degree because he did not follow all university regulations?

Appendix A
The Nuremberg Code—1947

What is now known as the Nuremberg Code was originally part of the court's decision during the International War Tribunal that charged Nazi physicians with war crimes. The text of this decision is given verbatim below.

Permissible Medical Experiments

The great weight of the evidence before us is to the effect that certain types of medical experiments on human beings, when kept within reasonably well-defined bounds, conform to the ethics of the medical profession generally. The protagonists of the practice of human experimentation justify their views on the basis that such experiments yield results for the good of society that are unprocurable by other methods or means of study. All agree, however, that certain basic principles must be observed in order to satisfy moral, ethical and legal concepts:

1. The voluntary consent of the human subject is absolutely essential. This means that the person involved should have legal capacity to give consent; should be so situated as to be able to exercise free power of choice, without the intervention of any element of force, fraud, deceit, duress, overreaching, or other ulterior form of constraint or coercion; and should have sufficient knowledge and comprehension of the elements of the subject matter involved as to enable him to make an understanding and enlightened decision. The latter element requires that before the acceptance of an affirmative decision by the experimental subject there should be made known to him the nature, duration, and purpose of the experiment; the method and means by which it is to be conducted; all inconveniences and hazards reasonably to be expected; and the effects upon his health or person which may possibly come from his participation in the experiment. The duty and responsibility for ascertaining the quality of the consent rest upon each individual who initiates, directs or engages in the experiment. It is a personal duty and responsibility which may not be delegated to another with impunity.

2. The experiment should be such as to yield fruitful results for the good of society, unprocurable by other methods or means of study, and not random and unnecessary in nature.

3. The experiment should be so designed and based on the results of animal experimentation and a knowledge of the natural history of the disease or other

problems under study that the anticipated results will justify the performance of the experiment.

4. The experiment should be so conducted as to avoid all unnecessary physical and mental suffering and injury.

5. No experiment should be conducted where there is an a priori reason to believe that death or disabling injury will occur; except perhaps, in those experiments where the experimental physicians also serve as subjects.

6. The degree of risk to be taken should never exceed that determined by the humanitarian importance of the problem to be solved by the experiment.

7. Proper preparations should be made and adequate facilities provided to protect the experimental subject against even remote possibilities of injury, disability, or death.

8. The experiment should be conducted only by scientifically qualified persons. The highest degree of skill and care should be required through all stages of the experiment of those who conduct or engage in the experiment.

9. During the course of the experiment the human subject should be at liberty to bring the experiment to an end if he has reached the physical or mental state where continuation of the experiment seems to him to be impossible.

10. During the course of the experiment the scientist in charge must be prepared to terminate the experiment at any stage, if he has probable cause to believe in the exercise of the good faith, superior skill and careful judgement required of him that a continuation of the experiment is likely to result in injury, disability, or death to the experimental subject.

See also George J. Annas, Michael Grodin, eds., *The Nazi Doctors and the Nuremberg Code* (New York: Oxford University Press, 1995).

Appendix B
The Declaration of Helsinki

The World Medical Association is an organization whose primary members are the national medical associations of each country. The association initially issued its statement on research ethics in 1964. It has been modified a few times. The declaration is primarily concerned with medical experimentation.

A. Introduction

1. The World Medical Association has developed the Declaration of Helsinki as a statement of ethical principles to provide guidance to physicians and other participants in medical research involving human subjects. Medical research involving human subjects includes research on identifiable human material or identifiable data.

2. It is the duty of the physician to promote and safeguard the health of the people. The physician's knowledge and conscience are dedicated to the fulfillment of this duty.

3. The Declaration of Geneva of the World Medical Association binds the physician with the words, "The health of my patient will be my first consideration," and the International Code of Medical Ethics declares that "A physician shall act only in the patient's interests when providing medical care which might have the effect of weakening the physical and mental condition of the patient."

4. Medical progress is based on research that ultimately must rest in part on experimentation involving human subjects.

5. In medical research on human subjects, considerations related to the well-being of the human subjects should take precedence over the interests of science and society.

6. The primary purpose of medical research involving human subjects is to improve prophylactic, diagnostic, and therapeutic procedures and the understanding of the aetiology and pathogenesis of disease. Even the best proven prophylactic, diagnostic, and therapeutic methods must continuously be challenged through research for their effectiveness, efficiency, accessibility, and quality.

7. In current medical practice and in medical research, most prophylactic, diagnostic, and therapeutic procedures involve risks and burdens.

8. Medical research is subject to ethical standards that promote respect for all human beings and protect their health and rights. Some research populations are

vulnerable and need special protection. The particular needs of the economically and medically disadvantaged must be recognized. Special attention is also required for those who cannot give or refuse consent for themselves, for those who may be subject to giving consent under duress, for those who will not benefit personally from the research and for those whom the research is combined with care.

9. Research investigators should be aware of the ethical, legal, and regulatory requirements for research on human subjects in their own countries as well as applicable international requirements. No national ethical, legal, or regulatory requirement should be allowed to reduce or eliminate any of the protections for human subjects set forth in this Declaration.

B.   Basic Principles for all Medical Research

10. It is the duty of the physician in medical research to protect the life, health, privacy, and dignity of the human subject.

11. Medical research involving human subjects must conform to generally accepted scientific principles, be based on a thorough knowledge of the scientific literature, other relevant sources of information, and on adequate laboratory and, where appropriate, animal experimentation.

12. Appropriate caution must be exercised in the conduct of research that may affect the environment, and the welfare of animals used for research must be respected.

13. The design and performance of each experimental procedure involving human subjects should be clearly formulated in an experimental protocol. This protocol should be submitted for consideration, comment, guidance, and where appropriate, approval to a specially appointed ethical review committee, which must be independent of the investigator, the sponsor or any other kind of undue influence. This independent committee should be in conformity with the laws and regulations of the country in which the research experiment is performed. The committee has the right to monitor ongoing trials. The researcher has the obligation to provide monitoring information to the committee, especially any serious adverse events. The researcher should also submit to the committee, for review, information regarding funding, sponsors, institutional affiliations, other potential conflicts of interest and incentives for subjects.

14. The research protocol should always contain a statement of the ethical considerations involved and should indicate that there is compliance with the principles enunciated in this Declaration.

15. Medical research involving human subjects should be conducted only by scientifically qualified persons and under the supervision of a clinically competent medical person. The responsibility for the human subject must always rest with a medically qualified person and never rest on the subject of the research, even though the subject has given consent.

16. Every medical research project involving human subjects should be preceded by careful assessment of predictable risks and burdens in comparison with foreseeable benefits to the subject or to others. This does not preclude the participation of healthy volunteers in medical research. The design of all studies should be publicly available.

17. Physicians should abstain from engaging in research projects involving human subjects unless they are confident that the risks involved have been adequately assessed and can be satisfactorily managed. Physicians should cease any investigation if the risks are found to outweigh the potential benefits or if there is conclusive proof of positive and beneficial results.

18. Medical research involving human subjects should only be conducted if the importance of the objective outweighs the inherent risks and burdens to the subject. This is especially important when the human subjects are healthy volunteers.

19. Medical research is only justified if there is a reasonable likelihood that the populations in which research is carried out stand to benefit from the results of the research.

20. The subjects must be volunteers and informed participants in the research project.

21. The right of research subjects to safeguard their integrity must always be respected. Every precaution should be taken to respect the privacy of the subject, the confidentiality of the patient's information and to minimize the impact of the study on the subjects' physical and mental integrity and on the personality of the subject.

22. In any research on human beings, each potential subject must be adequately informed of the aims, methods, sources of funding, any possible conflicts of interest, institutional affiliations of the researcher, the anticipated benefits and potential risks of the study and the discomfort it may entail. The subject should be informed of the right to abstain from participation in the study or to withdraw consent to participate at any time without reprisal. After ensuring that the subject has understood the information, the physician should then obtain the subject's freely-given informed consent, preferably in writing. If the consent cannot be obtained in writing, the non-written consent must be formally documented and witnessed.

23. When obtaining informed consent for the research project the physician should be particularly cautious if the subject is in a dependent relationship with the physician or may consent under duress. In that case the informed consent should be obtained by a well-informed physician who is not engaged in the investigation and who is completely independent of this relationship.

24. For a research subject who is legally incompetent, physically or mentally incapable of giving consent or is a legally incompetent minor, the investigator must obtain informed consent from the legally authorized representative in accordance with applicable law. These groups should not be included in research unless the research is necessary to promote the health of the population represented and this research cannot instead be performed on legally competent persons.

25. When a subject deemed legally incompetent, such as a minor child, is able to give assent to decisions about participation in research, the investigator must obtain that assent in addition to the consent of the legally authorized representative.

26. Research on individuals from whom it is not possible to obtain consent, including proxy or advance consent, should be done only if the physical/mental condition that prevents obtaining informed consent is a necessary characteristic of the research population. The specific reasons for involving research subjects with a condition that renders them unable to give informed consent should be stated in the experimental protocol for consideration and approval of the review committee. The protocol should state that consent to remain in the research should be obtained as soon as possible from the individual or a legally authorized surrogate.

27. Both authors and publishers have ethical obligations. In publication of the results of research, the investigators are obliged to preserve the accuracy of the results. Negative as well as positive results should be published or otherwise publicly available. Sources of funding, institutional affiliations and any possible conflicts of interest should be declared in the publication. Reports of experimentation not in accordance with the principles laid down in this Declaration should not be accepted for publication.

C.   Additional Principles for Medical Research Combined with Medical Care

28. The physician may combine medical research with medical care, only to the extent that the research is justified by its potential prophylactic, diagnostic or therapeutic value. When medical research is combined with medical care, additional standards apply to protect the patients who are research subjects.

29. The benefits, risks, burdens and effectiveness of a new method should be tested against those of the best current prophylactic, diagnostic, and therapeutic methods. This does not exclude the use of placebo, or no treatment, in studies where no proven prophylactic, diagnostic or therapeutic method exists. *Note of clarification on paragraph 29:* The W.M.A. is concerned that paragraph 29 of the revised Declaration of Helsinki (October 2000) has led to diverse interpretations and possible confusion. It hereby reaffirms its position that extreme care must be taken in making use of a placebo-controlled trial and that in general this methodology should only be used in the absence of existing proven therapy. However, a placebo-controlled trial may be ethically acceptable, even if proven therapy is available, under the following circumstances: (1) Where for compelling and scientifically sound methodological reasons its use is necessary to determine the efficacy or safety of a prophylactic, diagnostic or therapeutic method; or (2) Where a prophylactic, diagnostic or therapeutic method is being investigated for a minor condition and the patients who receive placebo will not be subject to any additional risk of serious or irreversible harm. All other provisions of the Declaration of Helsinki must be adhered to, especially the need for appropriate ethical and scientific review.

30. At the conclusion of the study, every patient entered into the study should be assured of access to the best proven prophylactic, diagnostic and therapeutic methods identified by the study.

31. The physician should fully inform the patient which aspects of the care are related to the research. The refusal of a patient to participate in a study must never interfere with the patient-physician relationship.

32. In the treatment of a patient, where proven prophylactic, diagnostic and therapeutic methods do not exist or have been ineffective, the physician, with informed consent from the patient, must be free to use unproven or new prophylactic, diagnostic and therapeutic measures, if in the physician's judgment it offers hope of saving life, re-establishing health or alleviating suffering. Where possible, these measures should be made the object of research, designed to evaluate their safety and efficacy. In all cases, new information should be recorded and, where appropriate, published. The other relevant guidelines of this Declaration should be followed.

Downloaded from the Web site of the World Medical Association: www.wma.net.

Glossary

advance directive   oral or written statements regarding the kind of medical care one wants in the future should one be unable to communicate.

arm of study   a course of involvement in a study; studies may have one or more arms; each arm may receive different kinds of treatment in order to make comparisons possible.

autonomy   the ability of human beings to make choices; the moral basis for informed consent in research.

beneficence   action taken in the interest of the subject; the moral basis for protecting subjects from undue risk.

blinding   in clinical trials, concealment of the nature of the intervention received by the subject; this may be single-blinding (the subject does not know) or double-blinding (neither the subject nor the researcher knows).

blinding   in publication, concealment of authorship when dealing with scientific reports and reviews.

case analysis   a method evaluating particular circumstances in light of generally accepted moral principles.

casuistry   a method of ethical analysis that involves applying general principles to individual cases, using clear-cut cases as points of comparison.

captive population   a group of people who are not entirely free to avoid unwanted attention or treatment.

cell lines   cells of a particular kind grown in the laboratory; these lines can replicate themselves indefinitely.

Centers for Disease Control and Prevention   an agency of the U.S. government that studies the incidence, frequency, and prevalence of disease and methods to control morbidity and mortality.

certificate of confidentiality   a protection given to some researchers that exempts them from certain obligations under civil and criminal law; for example, the duty to report observed crime.

Code of Federal Regulations   compilation of United States statutes.

compliance and **noncompliance**   conformity of subjects to the terms of a study, or failure to do so.

consent   expressed willingness, usually paired with *informed* to indicate a decision made in full knowledge of the nature and scope of available choices.

confidentiality   restriction of access to and use of information gathered in the course of research.

conflict of interest   the prospect of financial or other gain that could undermine fiduciary or professional judgment exercised to benefit others, not one's own self.

consequentialism   a method of ethical analysis that relies heavily on consequences (as against motives or the nature of actions) in order to evaluate the value of actions.

deception   actions taken in order to mislead; it may include outright lies or withholding of information.

deferred consent   consent sought after a course of action has been imposed on a person; usually applied to circumstances in which people are not capable of giving consent in advance because of an incapacity.

deontological ethics   a method of ethical analysis that relies heavily on the nature of duty (as against motives or consequences) in order to evaluate the value of actions.

embargo   in publication, withholding known information until a specified time.

ethics committee   a general term used to refer to committees having oversight of either clinical or research activities; see *institutional review board*.

equipoise   a state of indeterminacy about whether one drug or device is better than another; the moral basis for asking subjects to enroll in research.

exclusion criteria   factors that make people ineligible to join or to continue in studies.

exposure studies   studies that expose animals or humans to pathogens, injuries, or situations under controlled circumstances in order to study the effect of that exposure and/or a treatment.

framing effect   in psychology, the way in which presentation of information influences the way in which it is perceived and evaluated.

genetic therapy   therapy that involves alteration of the genetic make-up of an organism.

genome   a combination of the words "gene" and "chromosome"; refers to the entire genetic make-up of an organism.

germ-line intervention   a genetic intervention that affects not only the individual but can be passed along to offspring.

inclusion criteria   factors that make people eligible to join a study.

informed consent   a moral precept that requires disclosure of the nature and scope of a study to possible subjects; the process of making that disclosure.

institutional animal care and use committee   a committee that is charged to review and approve studies involving animals.

institutional review board (IRB)   a committee that is charged to review and approve studies involving human subjects; its primary charge is to protect the rights and welfare of subjects.

phase 1 studies   in government regulations, a study to evaluate the safety of a drug or device in humans; part of the process required to make a drug or device available to the public.

phase 2 studies   in government regulations, a study to evaluate the effect of a drug or device in humans; part of the process required to make a drug or device available to the public.

phase 3 studies   in government regulations, a study to evaluate the benefit of a drug or device in humans; part of the process required to make a drug or device available to the public.

phase 4 studies   in government regulations, a study to evaluate the effects of widespread use of a drug or device in humans after it is make available to the public.

randomization   the distribution by chance of subjects to the various arms of a study; intended to minimize possible bias.

recombinant DNA   a term used to refer to intentionally modified genetic sequences either in vitro or in vivo.

risk (minimal)   in government regulations, a term that refers to the probability that anticipated research risks are not greater than those encountered in daily life or during the performance of routine physical or psychological examinations or tests.

somatic cell nuclear transfer (SCNT) transplanting the nucleus of a somatic cell (not a gamete) into another cell which has had its nucleus removed, usually an ovum; this transfer is part of a process of inducing the new cell to behave as an embryo.

somatic treatment treatments that affect the body but do not alter the underlying genetic make-up of an organism.

subclinical markers laboratory evaluations to study the effect of medical interventions before the emergence of symptoms.

therapeutic research research believed to have some possible benefit for the subjects; the opposite of nontherapeutic research in which no benefit to the individual is foreseen.

vector in genetics, a mechanism by which a gene is delivered into an organism.

Cases by General Category

Aging and Longevity
Animal Research
Authorship, Publication, and the Media
Children
Clinical Care and Research
Conflicts of Interest
Deception
Genetic Research
Human Embryo and Fetus Research
Informed Consent
Institutional Review Boards
International Aspects of Research
Oversight
Placebos
Reproductive Research
Research Priorities
Social Uses of Research
Study Design
Subject Selection
Subjects' Rights and Duties
Tainted Data and Researchers
Transplantation
Vulnerable Populations
Women

Aging and Longevity

Cloning for Longer Life – 5.1
Curbing the Methuselah Vote – 5.12

Animal Research

Authorship, Publication, and the Media

Children

Clinical Care and Research

Conflicts of Interest

Deception

Genetic Research

Human Embryo and Fetus Research

Informed Consent

Institutional Review Boards

International Aspects of Research

Oversight

Placebos

Reproductive Research

Research Priorities

Social Uses of Research

Study Design

Subject Selection

Subjects' Rights and Duties

Tainted Data and Researchers

Transplantation

Vulnerable Populations

Women

Alphabetical List of Cases

Index